Running On Empty

How my wife and I overcame infertility

L. NATHANIEL

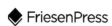 FriesenPress

Suite 300 - 990 Fort St
Victoria, BC, V8V 3K2
Canada

www.friesenpress.com

Copyright © 2016 by L. Nathaniel
First Edition — 2016

ISBN
978-1-4602-9796-4 (Hardcover)
978-1-4602-9797-1 (Paperback)
978-1-4602-9798-8 (eBook)

1. Biography & Autobiography, Personal Memoirs

Distributed to the trade by The Ingram Book Company

I would like to dedicate this book to my
partner: my faith, my Hope, my love

Introduction

MALE INFERTILITY ISSUES ARE DIFFICULT TO TALK about. Apart from the obvious fact that, for guys, fertility is tied up with ideas of potency and masculinity, infertility is also socially complex. It tests your relationships with your partner (if you have one) as well as your friends and family and perhaps even yourself and your sense for yourself as a man. These issues can be difficult to broach for the people who care about you.

It can be a tickly subject that seems as awkward to avoid as to address. Occasionally even the best intentions and encouragement of friends and loved ones fall flat or add to the discouragement. Sometimes it might almost be better to talk to a stranger about this stuff. Well that's me. You don't know me, but I've been through this.

If this is the boat you've found yourself in, you're not alone. Welcome aboard. If you've spent anytime exploring the decks, you probably know that the healthcare system can seem a contradictory labyrinth of uncertainty and reductionist interactions of what *should* be one of the most amazing experiences of your life. But there is another level to all of this, a deeper level of transformation to this story.

I decided to write this memoir for two reasons.

This was an important chapter in my life, and I felt that it might be interesting (or even instructive) to others facing similar issues. I wanted, on a practical level, to share the lessons I learned along the way, some tips on how to navigate health care and social systems, share the different options to family-making in theory and what we experienced in practice.

Perhaps more importantly, I wanted to elicit real hope in your heart of how, along this trip, I learned to transmute the deep challenges along the way into a stronger relationship with my partner[†], my friends and family, and ultimately myself, without losing my mind.

This is a memoir for those determined to build a loving family during their time on this planet, one way or another.

[†] For the purposes of this memoir, I will refer to my partner as Hope. This isn't her actual name, but it's certainly apt.

Vaclav Havel once said, "Hope is definitely not the same thing as optimism. It is not the conviction that something will turn out well, but the certainty that something makes sense, regardless of how it turns out."

I could not have put it better myself.

One

I AM INFERTILE.

For guys, there are many circumstances under which this can happen: sickness, injury, infirmity, and, of course, the congenital lottery of birth. For me it was the latter and faulty plumbing that meant I cannot produce sperm. And this is something I've known since I was a young lad and my mother broached the subject as part of "the talk." The point I am making here is that, for as long as I have known how babies are made, I've known that I wouldn't be making any that way.

However, *as* a guy, I concluded, a very long time ago, that to have no sperm is not really a big deal. Seriously. There's no love lost from zero spunk (a term for British readers). Heck, how could I miss something my body never had? I mean, it's not like I had it one day and then there was a poor quality assurance audit, a burst pipe, my body's sperm-making mechanisms suffering cata-strophic failure a-la British Petroleum's Deepwater Horizon—spill-ing out into a vast gulf of life-teeming oceans, ruining intricate ecosystems for everyone and everything else in the process. Nope. It's more like drilling for oil where there's no oil to be found. Except I ain't even waiting for the tumbleweed to blow past me in the background. Clearly the universe decided this body is so gorgeous—*yes, let's go with that*—that it didn't need tadpole-like gene bags hanging around in it.

"Go my child and live sperm-free!"

And so it is. Sperma de nada. No chance of any biologically linked offspring. Instead there is, how can I put this, a sea with no fish? A garden with no seeds? Everything *else*, however, is in perfect working order, and I am incredibly grateful for all of it, and have been every day of my life.

Well, every day of my life since *everything else* became an active ongoing concern. And alright, I wasn't always grateful. As anyone can imagine, growing up with a body that differs from what the media portrays as *normal* is obviously going to make anyone stop and think, *what's wrong with me?*

Kids, teenagers, and young adults tend to reflect on their differences, whether they be physical or otherwise, and often try to cover them up to fit in because that's how to stay connected to their community. Often such cover-ups are sustained by simple fear of rejection. However, for the most part, that's not how it was with me and *my* little difference growing up. In fact, because I knew I was different from a very early age, I developed this natural tendency to embrace my difference—and even be *thankful* that I was different.

Maybe it was a way to cope. Maybe it was a way to make myself feel special. Maybe it was a way to rationalize being the guy who was never going to be able to biologically procreate. I have to say, though, it really did not feel like a big deal for most of my childhood. Let's be honest, who actually thinks about having children while still a child themself?

Sure, we are bombarded with images of what a family looks like and what we should want when we grow up, but not in a deeply meaningful way. Growing up, did I think about the commitment, the responsibility, the nasty (or not so nasty) process of creating a child? Heck no! Of course, I wasn't bothered. Truth be told, most adults are barely bothered by such thoughts until they're facing them down, and that's something I was never going to have to do. For me, infertility meant even more chance to relax and not worry about unintentionally getting anyone pregnant. Not that I took much advantage of that fact—unfortunately this badge of honour did not automatically mean I was a chick-magnet.

Eventually adulthood helped me focus a bit more on my career and my life's vision and the early stages of where it was headed. University beckoned, and I wrapped myself up in the world of science, in biochemistry to be more specific. I convinced myself that the reason I had this condition was that I was going to be the one to discover what was wrong with me and how to cure it. What a noble quest for my ego to feast upon! However, once I discovered, after graduating, that this involved working in a laboratory three floors underground, unravelling DNA all day long in test tubes, and being cut off from sunlight, people and life—with the prospect of doing that every day for the next forty years—it just wasn't that alluring anymore. That was a significant breaking point.

I got really lost and confused at that point and had to accept that I would never understand why I was born this way or find a cure and that, fuck it, life was just too short to be missing out on all sorts of *other* things in the meantime. I decided I needed to start exploring the world and, through doing so, explore myself.

I was never very good with those messy things called feelings, though, particularly the difficult ones. So with this came the next rationalization—I was not *meant* for children, and so I was going to pursue the kind of intense, all-consuming, self-absorbed goals that only people who cannot have children are free to pursue. Well perhaps *some* parents could pursue them, I supposed, but they wouldn't be able to spend the kind of time with their kids that I would want to spend with mine if I could have them, which I couldn't. No judgment on them.

At that point in my life, I had conflated the idea of having a *family* with having *children*. I think it's important to note, that I think differently now.

Two

HAVING LIBERATED MYSELF FROM THE LAB, I FILLED my lungs with fresh air and decided to travel the world and tick all the experience boxes as I go. I was born, raised and educated in the West Midlands in the UK and, at nineteen, I hadn't seen much of the world. I'd create itineraries and set myself challenging tasks, all leading back to the ultimate goals of making it to all the continents in the world, meeting all sorts of people, and engaging different cultures and learning new ways of understanding society. I got pretty far with that I have to say. I didn't quite make it to Antarctica or the Arctic—they are just too bloody cold though ultimately I chose to settle in Canada instead. Don't ask

But I am getting ahead of myself.

I LEFT THE WEST MIDLANDS IN THE SUMMER OF 2002. I spent a long time in South East Asia. I worked and lived in Japan for two years to be precise. Living in Japan was like living on another planet. Of all the places I had the privilege of venturing, this place I found the most enigmatic, the most removed from what I had come to know about how the world works. I believe it had something to do with the fact that Japan had not opened its borders to foreign trade until 1868. All that time, an entire nation isolated to evolve in its own unique way. Japan was where my spirit really broke and also where I found myself more malleable to grappling life and what it means to be a human being.

Japan is made up of four main islands and thousands of smaller ones, and I lived on Shikoku, the smallest of the main ones. I was the only foreigner in town, and contrary to certain beliefs about how welcoming the society can be—and people there certainly *can* be—it was incredibly isolating. I like to call that period of my life painfully mind-broadening. I spent so much time with my own thoughts that I do believe I drove myself slightly nuts! I wasn't really thinking too much about the whole infertility thing, I was thinking more along other lines.

Who the hell am I? What am I going to do with my life? What do I want from this existence? Where do I fit in?

Now of course, I can see how all these quandaries are connected. However, at the time, with no answers and no one around me that I could understand well or could understand me—probably because I wasn't making myself very available—I needed to manage the overwhelming angst that came with this state. I do know plenty of folks who don't need to travel nine thousand miles to feel this way.

I lived in a very rural area of the country and would run to the top of the hill behind my apartment at 6:30 every morning and scream.

"You will not beat me!"

My poor neighbours likely thought, *crazy foreigner*. But heck, they gave me that blank undisguised look of bewilderment in the supermarket, the bank, the post office, and the movie theatre.

Some might revel in this, but for me, let's just say I never thought I'd see the day where I was empathizing with Tom Cruise. There is something very surreal about the experience of being stared at all day, *every* day, for literally two years that makes one question oneself. I don't know what it is. People would literally stop in their tracks, pause in-depth conversations, sometimes halt in the middle of the road—which was slightly worrying—just to stare until I got past.

The self-consciousness it induced was intense. After about six months, I would start gawking back to see if folks would stop. Nope! Succumbing to being overtly different was something, however, I had invited upon myself. No one was forcing me to live there. I will say this, though, it was vital in forcing me to recognize my inner uniqueness—I couldn't hide from it. Even though I knew people could not see who I was, the constant attention made me unbearably explicit to myself.

One thing it most definitely helped me do was open up a door to viewing how my own Western culture had impacted on forming my own identity. From how to be a man to being part of a community; from being successful, to being a good person in the world. It was only when I travelled to this place that I could really see what was at my core regardless of where I was, beyond culture, language, social constructs and history.

I took up running.

It felt like the only thing I could do to keep a sense of control and power in my life. What was surreal was that, for the first twenty-two years of my life, I could not run for more than two minutes. So I started to set myself goals and worked towards them and made them happen and, in doing so, achieved a sense of accomplishment. That was very important to my well-being. The multitude of parallels about running are too numerous to mention here. Suffice to say that running away from myself and the angst was the feeder of these victories!

I think I can safely say I took this process a step too far when I got down to forty kilograms. Part of the problem was I became so engrossed in literally running towards the goal of escaping self-acceptance that I would forget to eat a lot of the time. I was pretty lost running around trying to find myself again.

There were a few people I did actually manage to have superficial interactions with during my time in Japan. Grunts and passing eye locks with Japanese folks I worked with and other foreigners I met in different prefectures as I continued jumping around and around. Once I was done with Japan, Laos, China, Cambodia, Thailand, and South Korea, I eventually ran off to Australia, Africa North America, South America, and then back to Euro again.

Such a shame when I think back because I physically went to all these incredible places and met some profoundly intriguing people, but I was so checked out, disconnected, and alone that the folks who came across my path—who no doubt would have had so much to teach me about what I desired—were wasting their time. I do believe I met a lot of people during this time in my life, but my memory of these years is very limited because of the dissociation, and at the time, I was very grateful for this comfortable state.

Eventually I became so exhausted that I realized that who I was was going to need some serious reflection and work in order to be okay in the world—and I am not talking about the physicality of me, but the deeper stuff, the much deeper psychological stuff. Of course I was never going to admit that I needed help, so instead, I started training to become a mental health counsellor. You can see the logic right?!

This was a fascinating experience let me tell you.

I was so outside of my own body, so dissociated from people and circumstances, that neither of those two aspects would really affect me too much. As strange as it might sound—or maybe not if you've ever experienced this yourself—it felt safe and liberating to not be so interconnected to everyone and everything else around me. In a way it felt free. I felt like I was free from being asleep, acutely conscious of the influences of language and culture around me that would re-shape me into a certain expression of myself designed to fit in with the community. Of course the sacrifice of this "freedom" was abject loneliness. But I think I had already decided, based on my previous experiences, that this was an inevitable norm for me. Don't get me wrong, of course I still experienced being attracted to plenty of women, I just paid those feelings zero attention.

That went on for a couple of years. I barely spoke to anyone, and at one point was working four jobs at once. This surprisingly didn't pay as much as one might expect! Let this be a lesson to my own inner child: it is more prosperous to be in a peaceful state being who you *are* than in a highly anxious state being who you're *not*.

At times, I looked at children as products of their experience, blank slates awaiting the pens of fate. At other times I saw them as a conglomeration of genes waiting to be switched on and off depending on what their environment threw at them at a given age and how they interpreted the activity around and inside them. I have, of course, thought about what my children might have been like, my *biological* children. I think about what genes they might have inherited, what their personalities might have been like, their demeanours, their interests. I imagined what it would be like to see a potential mini version of myself, both in looks and in personality. What kind of ultimate mirror for oneself that might be like.

I came to appreciate that children are so sponge-like that there are pieces of oneself that can imprint on any child under the right conditions. And that thought has also transformed into how I might imprint on other people, particularly adults—and, of course, how other adults might imprint on me, and indeed how children might imprint on me. That is when I started to consider the possibility of what it is to be a parent. To be a guardian and guide for someone whilst they're trying to figure out who they are, how to be, and learning to become self-sufficient. I would say that becoming a counsellor helped me come to understand that we are all children and can be children of each other—and with each other—and that we are all connected. And yes, even connected biologically.

I remember watching a documentary about the history of the human race and the concept of the scientific Adam and Eve. It mapped out how we are all descendants of a community of human beings that originated in a now isolated village in Africa. It theorized that, at different points in time, when pieces of land were connected by ice, some of those people were bold, banished, or desperate enough to emigrate. Then the time-separated groups of those emigrated communities met up with each other later on in time, procreating to produce the diversity of human beings we have today. Well so far.

I have two main feelings about these kinds of theories. The first is that I often get suspicious of whoever is writing these theories and what their ultimate conclusion will be. For example, is the argument going to then be that a certain person is more evolved or advanced than the other—*oh look it just so happens to be the same type of person, biologically, as the theorist authoring this model.* And the second feeling is one of comfort and peace with the concept that we are all connected, and how at different points in time our ancestors thought, *I'm going for it!* and ventured out into the unknown. It seems to be a pretty common narrative in the lives of the thousands of people I've met over the years as a counsellor. I've also learned that everyone thinks that everyone else is normal and that they're *abnormal.* Well, based on the stats, it turns out that feeling abnormal is the norm. This might sound contrary, but rather than our sameness, it is our perceived differences in the experiences of ourselves that seem to be bridges that can connect us.

So back to my travels. Once I had reached what felt like the ends of the Earth—mainly because I weighed around forty kilograms and was running out of money—and had ticked the last main box I had on my list, which was to walk the Inca trail in Peru, I decided to return to base-camp also known as my mum's abode in England. Perhaps it's no coincidence that, along the trek to Machu Picchu, was a scattering of phallic symbols and ancient monuments honouring fertility. Pachamama, the female God of the mountain swarming with sheep and shepherds, reminded me of something. Oh yes, procreation. A reminder that Mother Nature has a way of bringing you full circle. Plus of course, I was more ready to hear her stubborn voice by then.

Upon returning to England and settling into a decent job, I starting to slowly reconnect with folks around me, making friends and getting healthier. As a man, I do believe I am socialized not to pay too much attention to feelings and to exert a sense of strength, authority, and control over my own life at least—particularly being raised in Britain. A friend of mine once considered whether someone can ever go back to reconnecting with their community once they have lived abroad because no one can completely relate to you in the new place because you engender foreign concepts, yet when you return, you cannot forget what you've learned from the place you went to live in and what it has taught you and challenged you about those concepts. Furthermore, whilst you've been away, everyone and everything has continued to evolve without you. Blimey! There must be a crap-load of ex-pats and folks who live abroad for a while before returning who could be an entire community unto themselves. If only they could sit still for five minutes!

The sense of disconnection continued along with the acute awakening to how sensitive I had become to social discourses. The thing about those bloody social discourses is that they can help folks come together—as well as, of course, control people's minds and behaviours en masse. But is that such a high a price to pay? I am, of course, being facetious—a perfectly healthy response to this predicament methinks.

Alcohol came into my life to help with the extreme social anxiety that was rapidly developing as a result of this situation. A sip here, a swig there just to take the edge off—it is incredibly effective, in the moment. Of course, those moments build up into days, weeks, and years. All of a sudden, these are not moments, this is your life. Some might say life is made up of moments. Each moment I could have chosen differently. Never underestimate the power of denial and a fragile ego. A fragile ego is a stubborn ass. I am fortunate enough to have had the social support around me to recognize that this was not going to turn out too pretty. People around me were, for the most part, supportive. It was me who was not able to accept myself.

If you are an infertile man—and perhaps the same might well be for an infertile woman—you might have asked yourself the question, *what's the point of my life*? At some point, many folks seem to think of where their life is headed and what legacy they might leave behind once they leave the physical realm of their existence on this planet. I had spent many years alone and focused on experiencing as much as possible as a loner, then focusing on a career and supporting others in ways I knew could be effective. My spirit needed fuel and needed to feel connected. I knew I was never going to be Mother Teresa. I craved physical intimacy too much!

I figured friendships and relationships, which I was not attracting into my life, were what I needed desperately. And like a magnet, they were never going to come as long as I repelled myself. I started to go to the doctor to explore how to get the best support possible, boost my body's health as much as I could, and feel better about myself in the process. I had suffered from sleep deprivation for around ten years and it was starting to take its toll on me mentally. As an aside, there is a great discourse around how parenting children enables us to parent ourselves, looking at self-discipline, forgiveness, learning and facilitating the journey of coming into oneself. I would say that this is also possible to do without children.

I was getting shingles and headaches, and as you can imagine, my moods were dark. That was another turning point for me. The doc I chatted with listened to my story and helped me come to terms with my condition. He had the most perplexed look on his face—kind of like a cross between three-day-old constipation and being asked to solve a quantum mechanics equation using only bananas. Yet at the same time, the words coming from his mouth were very reassuring and comforting. It was a bizarre experience. He also had with him a student doc listening in the corner to all of this which was a little disconcerting.

FYI, for anyone reading this, if you ever go to see a doctor or specialist of any kind and they have a student shadowing them, it is your basic human and legal right to ask them to leave if you are not comfortable. I'm talking about the student, of course, not the doc in this situation—although that would also be appropriate in some instances.

Three

ONCE I HAD FINALLY COME TO TERMS WITH MYSELF and reached the point where I was completely honest about everything, I did not care anymore about how others judged me. Well that's not strictly true, I *did* care, but I accepted the fact that I could not do anything about it. This was also the moment I started to be open to relationships. I had been on a few dates with a few girls, but it was not feeling very right. That's when Hope, the woman who would become my future wife, contacted me on the now all-powerful omnipresent social networking tool of Facebook.

But this was not that, not then anyway. This was in 2007, in the relatively early days when Facebook was first starting up. I barely used the site, and still don't. That she found me was actually pretty remarkable. But she did. She found me, noted my birthday on the profile I had created, and wished me a happy birthday. I was so naive I thought she had just *remembered* my birthday somehow.

You see, we had met each other chatting at a party whilst I was in Japan four years earlier and swapped contact details. She was one of those people I had grunted at superficially and bounced around, likely coming across as an utterly aloof git. This, for me, demonstrates not only what a lovely soul she has, but also the power of loving kindness and the diversity of human experience.

Amazingly enough I can recount a few memories of when I met her in Japan. Clearly, as far removed from myself I was, she left a lasting impression on me, one deep enough to be recalled consciously. Hope is a lovely and open-minded sensitive soul, and I felt very safe with her from the beginning. At this point in time I lived in Europe, and she lived in Canada. Not exactly round the corner, and I'm not the greatest swimmer in the world. However, within a year I'd flown to her, she'd flown to me, I'd flown back again, she'd flown back again. One of us had to make the decision to move. It was a no-brainer for me, to be frank. Canada, here I come!

I moved to Markham, Ontario, in the winter of 2009 and became a permanent resident in 2010. I want to acknowledge here that I recognize my privilege. I was white, was raised in an English-speaking country, relatively young, educated and—*guess what*—no children!

Settling in the Greater Toronto Area represented a new chapter in my life—a chance to start a new way of living, in a better headspace and within a sincere relationship that was both open and honest. Let me tell you, being in a relationship with someone you are one hundred percent yourself with—and who knows everything about you—is a very calming experience. I recognized how much time I was wasting trying to be something else with others and why I was attracting the wrong people for me. They were likely doing the same thing for themselves and attracting an insincere me. All for good intentions, of course, but ultimately incredibly unhealthy and unhelpful.

Buying a house and getting married, life looked a lot like success to me. During this time, the discussion about children finally reappeared again in my life. Children. I had not thought about it again until this point. Children. Neither of us were sure at this point what or whether we wanted or would have them. Children. We read a lot, talked a lot to others and each other. Children. Eventually we signed up for a twelve-week course for folks who could not have children biologically. These were mainly same-sex couples, and it was good to be invited into this other community where folks had also known for different reasons that they were going to need medical or social service intervention to have children of their own.

I met some amazing people and formed meaningful friendships there, and for that I am grateful. I would highly recommend attending support groups for folks experiencing the same issues as you. It is a great source of strength and validation to discuss issues that others might not be able to relate to and spend time with folks who can appreciate the ever present background hum of issues like infertility. One of the exercises we did was to get into sub groups and deduce where we were at in the decision-making process for questions like: Have you decided whether to have children? Have you decided whether you want to try IVF or IUI? Have you considered adoption? We had to insist on the creation of a new category called *dunno yet*.

Later in the course, I recall a presentation on sperm and egg donation, and the chat Hope and I had about how difficult it would be to conceive (ha!) of using another man's sperm. Let me burst that illusory bubble—as soon as the booklet of sample donor profiles was passed around the room the first page was opened and much like a child in a candy store we exclaimed: "I want that one!" Apparently the fact that he had two eyes a nose and a mouth was similar enough for us to feel like we could relate to this donor. It was a very special moment, although she did share she liked the person's character from his essay to the potential recipients.

Looking back, that was the spark that ignited the fire that would propel us on our journey to exploring reality with theory. It was not until that moment that we could actually visualize the possibility of flicking through books, leaflets, catalogues. Asking ourselves profound questions like *why do we prefer this profile to that profile?* and *does it matter?*

Before this, I would say that our soap boxes were numerous. For example, in order to become a donor, these folks have to take a battery of extensive tests to be considered compliant—or rather to have their *stuff* considered compliant. Medical histories, IQ tests, physical and emotional assessments, personality and psychological inventories—all this is just for the privilege of enjoying oneself for two minutes in a locked room. We haven't even gotten to the analysis of the actual swimmers yet. One can't help but wonder how many of us may not be alive if our forefathers had had to go through similar scrutiny.

Clearly we did not decide that very night on the spot, but for our circumstances, the sperm donation certainly opened a door we had never even been sure existed until that evening.

What can be incredibly off-putting, if you're not prepared for it, is the business-like nature of sperm and egg banks. This was not only our experience with the industry, but also the experience of others I have spoken with. It is on the cusp of being a healthcare institution and a private franchise. Canadian donors do not actually get *paid* for donating, hence the much higher rate of American donors.

A large proportion of donors are young white men who could do with the money, or not, but want it anyway, as young white men tend to. You might think that it cannot be that expensive to store a relatively inexpensive (or altogether free) commodity that is incredibly small in physical size. And in truth it's not the storage that is expensive. The process of shipping it from sperm bank to clinic, to taking it out of the box, to washing it, to testing it, to analyzing the results, to writing down the results, to showing you the results, to explaining what the results mean, to actually then going ahead with exploring the various options involved in putting the stuff into someone's body—well, all this adds up. All for the privilege of actually knowing whose "stuff" you are receiving-well it is anonymous, but open for potential off-spring to meet should they wish to.

The gentleman from the sperm bank was sporting a classic spray tan look. He wore a Calvin Klein suit, travelled with state-of-the-art Mac laptop, had a gourmet coffee to go in one hand, and a leather bag in the other. Clearly they were not struggling for clients. I will be the first to admit I am a proud cynic when it comes to salespeople. I can always feel a part of my brain check out as soon as I hear the special cold call telephone ring, the doorbell chime, or the overly-excited advert audio. I guess I can appreciate that it is a niche that many of us cannot do too much about. They have you literally by the balls. That is where it has similarities to the healthcare system. I cannot gain access to the medication or services I have needed in my life without the help of willing providers—and I am a white, male, English-speaking, employed, housed, supported, straight citizen of the world aka super-privileged.

Then there was adoption to consider.

An adoption agency had come to speak to the group along with a couple who had adopted two children. They were not beating around any bushes when they told us that their daughter had tried to set fire to one of her adoptive parents' hair, and their son had burned a thousand ants on the coal fire on a weekly basis for years.

"We want you to think seriously about this before you embark on what it entails."

Yup, got the message, a child is for life, not just for Christmas!

Adopting children, although profoundly different in its process to the sperm donor route, prompted us to explore similar philosophical and self-analytical quandaries.

Neither of us are black, how would we feel adopting a black child? What about a child who had been abused? A child with mental health issues, physical abnormalities, fetal alcohol syndrome, siblings? What about a child whose biological parents want to keep in touch with them?

I have always been a pretty autonomous fellow. Whenever I meet someone for the first time, I accept the fact that they come with a history beyond my control, one that I had no part in. It's a bit like dating, and so I can always make my own independent decisions whether to pursue that relationship or not—and vice versa for the same reasons. But adoption is sticky, for the stakes are higher. How on Earth can I possibly know whether I will be the right person for this child and the pre-existing issues they need particular nurturing around? Both the known and unknown ones.

Of course, you wouldn't know all the unforeseeable issues of your own biological children either—it is simply the timeframe at which you know them, e.g., before they're in your life or afterward. It made me stop and think, *how can I possibly know whether I have the skills to support them in the way they need?* Both adopted children and biological children. These questions were certainly a sobering experience for me. I have enough issues of my own, and a child—who did not choose me for a father—would be exposed to them and the history I came with for goodness sake! Perhaps in a parallel universe there are a bunch of children in care making decisions about which adoptive parents they are going to choose. Flicking through catalogues of potential parents with photo-shopped side profiles of them hugging each other over a sunset backdrop, conveniently hiding their deep-seated anxieties that lie dormant just waiting to be unleashed upon the unsuspecting pre-pubescent.

"Yes, well, I'll have *those two!*"

After the end of the course, we decided to explore this option a little more. We went through another assessment with our local adoptive agency and saw fit to attend one of their mandated education sessions before being allowed to be added to the pile of prospective guardians. Run by two social workers, they explained the process of waiting three years, then being attached to a social worker who would then assess us, get to know us over a period of many months, understand our personalities, our hopes for children, what we had in terms of child-rearing competencies, our backgrounds, psychological make-up, favourite flavours of ice cream, zodiac signs, and how many months before we stopped wetting the bed. At that point it is the social worker who would be evaluating, based on this information and the information regarding the children in the adoption agency's basket of children, who would be most appropriate.

That is not to say we would have no say. A self-assessment needed to be filled in first. I thought I was a relatively open-minded guy until the questions were staring at me in the face in black and white:

Would you take a child with a terminal illness; with a biochemical deficiency; with profound life-long mental illness... to name a few.

When I painted a picture of myself with this knowledge, fear-consuming feelings boiled up followed by humiliation of my frightened little ego. I really was not as loving and accepting as I would like to see myself as. That was a hard reality check and a deep process to be okay with—accepting I'm just not as decent of a person as I thought I was. I realized that, for myself at least, there was a profound difference between coming to terms with the knowledge that a child that you had supported from birth came to have these diagnoses, and knowing about their existence prior to having any relationship with them. Somehow I felt that, in a situation like the former, I would be devastated but would consider it something I would process, learn to understand and give my all to developing the necessary skills and resource-tapping needed to support them. Yet with a situation like the latter, there is somehow a moment of choice. A moment to stop and think whether I want to choose to embrace these experiences as part of becoming a parent.

It made me recognize that life had been survivable because I didn't have to know everything all at once. In not knowing everything that was coming all at once, I had been able to take circumstances one day at a time, one hour at a time in some instances. I suspect that there is only so much the human mind can take in at once and hope to adjust to. Mind you, at the moment of putting down our names to be on the adoption wait list, we were informed it would be three years before we would hear *anything* about next steps anyways, so I guess we did have time to reflect on all possibilities.

There is something very seductive about the belief that by being there with your child *from birth* you can somehow control who and what they might become and what they will be exposed to—somehow selecting what life dishes out for them. What rubbish.

There is a big part of me that laughs at this idea and judges it as incredibly ignorant. Yet I will fully admit there is another part of me that embraces the supposition that somehow loving a child enough from the first moments of life will protect them from those elements of their destiny you do not want them to experience. Let me tell you, if there is anything I am learning from this whole children malarkey, it is that, as a person who cannot just bonk and hope for the best, it is more about knowing who you are. If you know who and what you really are as a human being and are okay with all your own faults and frailties, then you can look at your potential child in the eyes and say, "I love you."

Because what you are simultaneously saying is "I love myself enough to believe I can love you right," warts and all!

ANYWAY, HOPE AND I WERE MARRIED IN AUGUST OF 2012, and that was, of course, after we had the distraction of buying a house the year before . And during this time, the prospect of children was like a white noise in the background, something that just felt would be not going away. The home-seeking was an arduous process; however, we knew we wanted three bedrooms. There was no denying that the hopes of having children—plural— became central in every decision-making process. From an early age I had always looked forward to the day that I would be paying mortgage instalments. I was a pretty insecure child, adolescent, and adult, and as a result had wanted to take charge of my life as early as I could. Being a home-owner was a major goal for me— embracing my sense of *home*.

I had spent a lot of my life, since leaving school, working and travelling all over the world looking for a place I could feel settled.

I realized during my travels that what I was seeking was a way to feel settled in myself. Now that I was feeling secure in a loving relationship, I was allowing myself to calm down somewhat. But old habits die hard, and being used to the anxious energy, it felt wrong not to keep moving. So my outlets included intense exercise and deep focus in my work-life.

As a trained mental health counsellor, I would say my behaviour seemed akin to being traumatized. I knew it was not necessary for me to feel anxious. I was housed, employed, had a social support network, and was physically healthy. But every day felt like a carbon copy of the last. I felt desperately lonely and bored within myself. Do not misunderstand. I love Hope very much. I do think it is quite possible to be lonely in oneself and one's life and be in a healthy loving relationship at the same time. I see it in terms of interdependence. I did not depend on my partner to be my sole source of comfort and respite from life's frustrations. I never felt the need or drive to put that responsibility onto her. No, it was my responsibility to recognize, acknowledge, and respond to my own inner struggles. Hope was my confidant—my sounding board—and I was and am incredibly grateful to have that in my life. She would encourage me to pursue hobbies and personal interests. I joined groups, art classes, trained for a marathon, and tried to push myself to go out with new friends.

However, I noticed myself becoming depressed. I did not handle large groups of people too well. I would find the superficial conversations—which are inevitable in large group dynamics—pointless and boring. That theme kept coming up. Boring. In fact, I managed to uncover diaries I had kept during my early childhood years and that was a common feeling I wrote: *Boorrriiiing*. I struggled with this feeling a lot clearly. I do know that my mother had always had a low boredom threshold herself, and she had had four children with no support!

During the three years since moving countries to be with Hope, I had changed jobs four times—well three really (the one job evolved into another role without my choice). Hope would say I should include the three-day stint at a part time job I had in the kitchens in a long-term care facility when I first moved whilst looking for something more permanent. By the end of the third year, I was back onto employment sites seeking something new to aspire to become or achieve. I was bored. Bored with life. I would reflect back on different stages of my life (I was still a young man) and sometimes say to myself, *Jesus, am I really still alive?!*

Now, this might be something that many men go through. I've heard it called a quarter-life crisis. What I was very cognizant of, though, was to question myself about whether I was pursuing children now in the hopes that the experience would bring me a more fulfilling an enriching life. I pondered on this for some time. My initial reaction was that it would not be wise to have children to fill this hole in my life. My second contrary reaction was to question why the heck *isn't* that a good reason to have children? Of course, it is going to bring an added dimensional depth to your life experience. Isn't that an incredibly good reason to have children? Isn't that why we choose to embark on just about anything? Isn't it with the hope that it will make us better people? That it will help us learn more about ourselves, what we're capable of, and how to overcome challenges and enjoy the precious loving moments in the process?

Four

SO THERE WE WERE, HOMEOWNERS MARRIED FOR about six months. That's when we decided to try to have a child. The major pieces were in place in my mind. It felt like the groundwork had been responsibly laid. We had a home with plenty of space, near a school. We had safety, opportunity, and social supports. There was a life-insurance policy, secure employment, and time for self-reflection and mutual support in the relationship. Surely we were ready.

It had been a year and a couple of months since finishing off the parenting course for folks who cannot conceive on their own. We had opted to preliminarily approach a fertility clinic that some of our new found friends had been through and had success with. I imagine that this is similar to most if not all fertility clinics at least in Canada. The process was to initially meet with the doctor to discuss our case before monitoring the menstrual cycle. The purpose of this was to make sure that everything was in good working order and determine when would be the optimum time to try for fertilization.

OKAY GUYS, CONSIDER THIS AS IUI 101.

IUI stands for Intra-Uterine Insemination. That means attempting to fertilize the egg inside the body. That involves the sperm being donated, going through a battery of tests and cleansing, and then put in a special syringe designed to get as close as possible to the opening of the uterus for the sperm to get more of a head-start than they would without intervention.

The other method used in fertility clinics is IVF [in vitro fertilization]. That is when the egg is extracted from the body and both the sperm and egg are introduced to each other in a petri dish and—once fertilization is successful—selectively planted back into the uterus to (hopefully) attach to the lining and, *presto*, preggers.

WE OPTED FOR IUI. FIRST OF ALL, WE PRESUMED that Hope had no fertility issues of her own. Second, it's incredibly expensive to do IVF—not that IUI is cheap, it isn't—so IUI it was. For those of you who want figures, it ranged between $15,000 to $20,000 total to do IVF-that is including, procedures, medications, other services necessary and possibly more, depending on your situation. IUI is around $1500 a shot to wash and prep and inseminate-that is not including drugs or whether you need to buy sperm from somewhere, or several other fees depending on your situation or clinic.

When we started to deliberate on when to give it our first shot, I kept imagining the countless potential beings which could result from our choice of that particular donor, and that particular deposit he made on that particular day, and then ending up with only eleven million sperm (the estimated count our first attempt had). It's pretty crazily mind-blowing that then the choice to do it

one month instead of the next would produce a completely different combination of genes and completely different set of potentially billions of people. It's truly nuts when I think about it.

The process of choosing a donor had been made. We liked to
think that we had some kind of criteria, but really, it could have
been any number of donors that we did not know. The biographies
were brief, and the pictures all blurred into one faceless male.
Caucasian, blue eyes, slim, young, smiling. It was like looking at
the Hollywood A-list, which is to say kinda boring, superficial,
and meaningless. It also served as a reminder that these are the
very categories to which I myself am assigned and that we live
in a world that sees fit to grant me privileges based on those
categories. You might be surprised to hear that it brought up a
lot of anxious thoughts about bringing a child into a world full of
sexism, racism, homophobia, classism and general hatred for difference and an eagerness for conformity. So we kept reminding
ourselves that, although a lot of attention is paid to these aspects
of humanity, there is also plenty of love, compassion, understanding and collaborative networks too. Being in a loving relationship
helps cultivate that and remind me how much harder it is to do
alone—and that's coming from a privileged straight white man.
Just saying.

We tried to be patient to accommodate both of us being in a
good headspace and a good physical space within our lives.
However, the self-induced pressure of being not in our twenties
by this point certainly propelled us to try a little quicker than we
might have otherwise wanted to. Everybody's circumstances are
different. Our circumstances were that one of us was out of work,
and we had just bought a house. We were going to a transitional
time, I was changing jobs, and Hope was making long-term life-
changing decisions. Someone else might find some other pressure

to manage as they try to determine when to go for it. Moving homes, dying parents, relationship issues, money worries, health concerns—you name it. There does seem to be one indisputable fact in life, though: that it is in constant change. Change on a micro scale some days. Other days it is on a macro scale, but it is always in flux. So navigating that fluidity and trying to determine such a profound change alongside consistent emerging change is an individual decision for everyone. Of course, this does not just limit itself to making a child.

However, let me mention here what kind of place we were in. One of the commitments to going through IUI is the need to monitor the ovulation cycle. This involved getting up several times a week, taking Hope to the clinic, having invasive procedures done, on a full bladder, by someone we had never met with minimal interaction, followed by being pricked for a blood test. At the time, we were conscious about finding the time to do this when we both found jobs. So the decision was that we would launch operations during a window of time when I had three weeks in between jobs. That's when we would go for it.

This was in February 2013.

Maybe it was the stress that prevented it working. Maybe it was the pressure of getting up so early and being invaded in a way that Hope had never been before by a stranger. Or maybe it was the $900 worth of drugs we "chose" to pump into Hope to delay ovulation because the day turned out to be a workday for her. Yes, when someone is in an unusual situation, instead of calling in sick or explaining that one has a doctor's appointment, that's what we chose instead. Nine hundred dollars so we could delay ovulation by one day and try one day later, a Saturday instead.

Let me emphatically encourage anyone here who might be going through the same experience, if any healthcare provider comes at you with a needle, to ask, at the very least, two questions first.

"What is that, and how much is it going to cost?"

We didn't ask, and so we didn't know it would cost $900 total until *after* the healthcare provider stuck it into Hope, nor were we informed that she would need two more doses which were to be self-administered. In my opinion this was rather poor practice and incredibly presumptuous. There are folks out there that would simply not be able to afford that, and had we known up front it would have sobered us up enough to decide to wait until the following month and wake up to the ridiculousness of what we were doing by putting work before potential family.

It never ceases to amaze me how these clinics—any health centre for that matter—can so often seem to forget they are dealing with people in vulnerable states. And when people are in vulnerable states, they need extra support, extra education, extra time, extra communicative staff. And the laughable circumstance of it all is that often these environments are set up to inevitably create staff behaviours that are distant and disconnected, educated on an a need to know basis, stretched for time, aggravated, frustrated, and stressed, and lacking the energy, time, or will left to give anything of themselves to relay back to the person what is happening. That is where self-education, self-support and self-management skills are crucial. I have certainly learned that I can never learn enough how to cultivate these.

It was February 9th 2013, the morning of our first insemination attempt. The roads were quiet, the street lights were still lit up, and the sky was black. This might not sound like an ideal moment to recall for such a time, but both Hope and I *love* this kind of atmosphere and find it very comforting. I think it is safe to say we are both introverts. We drove over to the clinic, which took around thirty minutes each way in good traffic. We parked the car, which of course was not free, and there was a time-limit on how long we could park.

At the clinic, we were handed a consent form to agree to not sue them if the child turned out to be deformed, mentally retarded, or left-handed or prefer blue to pink. We promised not to. The confidentiality standard of the clinic was not exactly over-rated. All people attempting to use their services to get pregnant had to write their names on a list in order of entry into the clinic, along with their cycle day, for everyone to see. I kept looking to see if Mickey Mouse was on day 100 as a proverbial fuck you, but alas folks were compliant. Yep, this certainly is a niche, and people know their choices are limited.

One blood test and a consent form photocopy request later, and we were told to wait two hours before the unit of sperm we ordered could be thawed and the staff would be ready to carry out the procedure. Of course that turned out to be three and-a-half hours, involving re-parking the car and paying the difference. Heck, I suppose it gave us something to do! Some people might consider that time a great moment to reflect and prepare. However, we had already done that for the last year. We were bored shitless after twenty minutes!

Eventually, the time came for us to go into a waiting room, i.e. the room where the procedure would happen. By this point it was approaching lunch time, and we were both pretty hungry. We were feeling high, however, on the situation and eager to get it done. So Hope prepared herself physically and mentally. There was a knock on the door, and in walked a busy nurse with a serious look on her face—this person was on a mission! Holding the tube that contained the swimmers, freshly washed and centrifuged, and ready for their final journey, she quickly yet methodically assumed the position.

Although we were initially told it would not be permissible, the nurse who carried out the procedure allowed me to push the syringe to send the swimmers on their way. And it some small way, that did kind of feel like an attempt to involve me in the process, which I know Hope certainly appreciated. So please note, if any health provider denies you the right to push that syringe, please challenge it.

The actual procedure of watching Hope feel uncomfortable yet managing it well as the speculum was introduced, followed by the sperm being injected into her, lasted about two minutes in all. We were then given fifteen minutes alone in the room to digest what had just happened and get ready to get out!

And there it was. Done.

We spent a couple of minutes smiling at each other, and I could sense Hope's vulnerability and a sense of *no going back now* came over us. She asked me talk to her tummy and pray over it to support the process as much as possible. I stroked her head in a comforting way, which she soon begged me to stop due to the itchiness it induced. We started to look around the room and there were large pictorial diagrams of the ovulation and fertilization cycles. Hope asked me to talk her through them, and as I did so, drawing on my rudimentary gynecological knowledge, we started to re-live, in our own minds, what our potential egg-turned-child had gone through to get here. We were blown away as we thought about it again and again—the odds, the battles, the journey every we had to go through with the clinic and negotiating our own relationship to the IUI process, and finally what these sperm and this egg had done simultaneously. There was a moment of connected empathy between the macro and microscopic level, and it was a very peaceful and profound moment...

...followed by a sharp shift in focus as our fifteen minutes was up.

We were informed that another blood test would be needed in two weeks *on the dot* to confirm whether we had a pregnancy or not. And let me tell you, *that* waiting game was a whole new ball of wax!

IT SURPRISES ME AS I WRITE THIS, BUT WE STARTED watching all sorts of documentaries and videos about the Law of Attraction. Basically, our attempt to feed into the illusion that we had any kind of control over the chances of it working. At that time, the so-called Law of Attraction was a trendy wave sweeping the internet and chat show circuit. Its premise is that one's state of mind of believing something will happen or *is* happening will increase the likelihood of it happening. Do not misunderstand, there is an element of this philosophy I believe in whole-heartedly. Mainly the bit that discusses how really no one knows anything, so you might as well try and feel as positive as you can about life as it tends to be a more pleasant experience... *that* bit! It is not easy at times; however, I have always strived to be a guy who counts his blessings. And I am very blessed.

Every day involved waking up and praying to the universe, mentally picturing positive vibes radiating from our minds and bodies to the outside world. Inviting the pulsating good energy fields from anywhere we could experience and believing that they would ripple across from those other areas of our lives and the lives of others around us to focus in and positively affect this process of getting pregnant. Day three.

Day four.

Day five.

Hope and I were very aware that the placebo affect was going to engulf us, and we bit every hook it gave us! Law of Attraction, baby! Every symptom that Hope thought she might be having, we took as a sign with gratitude, every mention of children around us, we took that as a portent. Thank you very much. Day six.

Day seven.

Day eight.

At this point we had formed good friendships with a few couples from the course we had embarked on a few months earlier. And we knew that some of them were already pregnant. We took that as a positive sign. Heck, we even took the fact that I had been fired and rehired as a sign! And of course, we had every symptom you could think of, sweat, tummy pain, waking in the night, munchies... yep we took full advantage of *that* one, even she did! Day nine.

Day ten.

Day eleven.

By now there had not been any sign of the next period, which we took as the ultimate sign that this was it, this was going to happen for us. Day twelve.

Day thirteen.

Day fourteen: blood test day.

WE HAD DECIDED NOT TO TAUNT OURSELVES WITH pregnancy tests although I can tell you now that we know people who found out they were pregnant through a Dollar Store test. So bear that mind if you are considering it and you see the plethora of tests ranging from a few bucks to closer to a hundred. The Dollar Store is your place.

We had decided visit one of our close friends immediately after the blood test—they had just given birth to their first baby. It just seemed fitting at the time. So another trip to the clinic, another vial of Hope's blood, and off we went up the highway to see another couple's newborn. Anxiously awaiting the phone call, we stopped off at a local mall to just walk around and keep ourselves distracted and ready for when that call came.

It came while we were in a food court. How romantic.

It was Hope's phone they called, and she knew immediately it was them without seeing the number. All I could see was the look in her beautiful brown eyes as she held the phone to her ear and a great grey sadness came over her like cold London smog in early winter. I could feel myself dissociate and shift straight into comfort mode.

She hung up the phone once it was done and repeated what she was just told.

"It didn't work. I'm not pregnant."

"It's okay, hon."

I took her hands, and she stared over my shoulder for a moment as if momentarily distracted, trying to absorbed everything that had happened. I tried to imagine what it must have been like for her, having so many invasive procedures and managing the discomfort of numerous technician strangers and nurses prod her and poke her.

After about a minute, which felt more like an endless moment, she started to well up. Now, as strange as this sounds, I took this to be a good thing. I saw it as a plus because it meant that she would not hold it all in. She would be able to live through this moment and move past it by mourning the disappointment and burst baby bubble we had dreamed up for ourselves in the weeks leading up to this moment. We spent about another half an hour in silence and tears absorbing the feelings while in a food court, surrounded by families with their children.

Again, I actually think this was a good thing—no, I am not a sadist—for it meant that we were surrounded by hope and an image of what could be. The ultimate message of the push–pull process of attempting to create life is that there is, at least whilst your partner is still menstruating, hope. And hope has gotten a lot of people through a lot of tragedies and disappointments over the course of human history. And there we were, in a food court, our disappointment a mote of sadness caught in the florescent lights and dry recycled air of a busy shopping centre.

We would have to turn to hope to feed our dream and re-energize ourselves in order to move forward. This was only a first attempt. There would be others.

Five

WHAT DO YOU DO TO PICK YOURSELF UP AFTER A DIS-
appointment? I tend to go running or go for a walk. Either way, I
need to move.

But this was February, the dead of winter. Canada. So unfortunately, movement was restricted. There were also other minor
background stressors in our lives. In the fall, I had decided to take
a risk and switch careers. It was actually initially a test of change,
moving from mental health counselling to quality improvement
in health care systems. I had gotten tired of supporting people
only to witness the system around them fail and occasioning
the re-unravelling of their lives. In other words, the system to
me was perfectly designed to achieve the rather spotty results it
was getting, and so I felt compelled that, somehow, I would try
to improve things. I found a permanent position and took it, only
to find that, four weeks later, the government was deciding to
axe the entire agency that had been there for years—did not see
that coming!

The decision from on high was to move all our roles into a different agency and ask us to reapply for them. For some curious and
unknown reason, the universe conspired to help me reacquire my
job, whilst the rest of my colleagues, some who had been there for

years, were unsuccessful and no longer employed! I did not actually know that I had managed to stay employed until the very end of January. A month before we tried that first time.

Now I am a firm believer that mental health and wellbeing is truly the root of most if not all physical ailments. At the very least it is, to my mind, a major contributor. As soon as I knew that I had kept my job, I became very ill with terrible symptoms and exhaustion—what some folks might call the man-flu. This was during the short gap between my job at the redundant agency and my job at the new agency. Again, that was when we had tried to time the first try. Hope too was trying to establish herself in a new job. There was, in other words, a great deal of non-fertility-related stress, which contributed to some crazy decisions. For example, when we found out that the insemination day was a Friday, rather than take a sick day, we pumped her full of incredibly expensive drugs to delay her ovulation until the weekend. Crazy, right? That is what anxiety and stress do to people. It makes them crazy and screws with their judgement.

We tried to tell ourselves that it had not been the right time. But we were relieved that we had at least tried. The way I approach a challenge is to try, try, and try again. Try different approaches, and come back to approaches that have moved you nearer to your goal in some way. Pace yourself, stay patient, but keep persistent. You may even be relieved, in a way, that it had not worked if you have felt that, with the angst energy going into the process, the outcome would likely have absorbed that negative energy. Put it this way, if someone is in a shitty mood and they make you dinner, do you think they are going to produce a masterpiece of delicately poached salmon or something more akin to frozen fish sticks? I think it is safe to say we were seeing it as a dry run!

If you have had at least one experience of this already, then you'll know how incredibly expensive this process is. It cost us a total of around $3500, so, naturally, we could not afford to just try the next month without some planning. However, the nurses were not particularly cognizant of this and explicitly expected us to continue trying immediately. Chance would be a fine thing, and money would be an even finer thing! And so it went for the next six months. Save, work, save, work, save, work. Meanwhile at work, people who knew that Hope and I were *trying* without knowing the issues we were facing and the route that those issues were forcing us to follow were happily chiming in on the subject.

"At least you get to have lots of sex!"

All well-meaning support, of course. Winking, elbow nudging, wry smiles and the occasional double entendre.

My response was a quiet smile and a ready supply of alternate conversational subjects. It is truly amazing to me how free some people feel to investigate the sex lives of others once they know that baby-making is on the agenda, such as asking someone when they stopped using protection. There may be other types of unsolicited comments and questions new parents are bombarded with, especially if they are same-sex parents, or racially distinct from their baby, or part of a more complicated arrangement of some kind. I had many hazy daydreamy moments of how I might best articulate a response to well-meaning but intrusive comments of friends and co-workers. Most of them included the phrase *why don't you fuck off* or some slight linguistic variation thereof. But that really is not helpful for anyone now is it? Well, that's not *completely* true; it's very helpful for stress relief in the moment for me! But I am not suggesting you do that.

We did not know exactly when we were going to give it a second shot. I called the adoption agency again just to make sure we were still on their list.

"Yes you are. You have been on here for a year, so only two more years to go."

Gee, thanks.

It was surreal to think that, if we were to end up adopting, our eventual child was actually alive at that moment and that we might be walking past them in the mall, on the street, in the supermarket. It made me think about time differently and how events are already unfolding as they should, and that took a little bit of the pressure off and relieved to urge to try and be in control of things beyond my control.

Living in the first world, saving up for our second attempt was about daily habits for us. I was biking to work an hour and a half each day and making all meals daily. Occasionally we would spoil ourselves to a dinner out when we spotted a two-for-one deal at a cheap Chinese buffet. We rented free movies and documentaries from the local library. We walked a lot in the mornings to watch the sunrise and to help us stay grounded. We read stories to each other and made up stories and played board games and made up games and window shopped and took forest walks—our lives were about saving money and staying happy and healthy.

In a way, our situation was bringing us closer than ever and helping us get through some difficult times. We were going through a lot of other experiences at the same time that I have not mentioned here. We were focusing on saving, and we were working as a team and getting to know each other in a way that was authentic—who we really are beyond all the glitter and gold—gaining an understanding of the core ingredients that actually made up our relationship. It was actually quite a magical time, and I do believe, for a first year of marriage, a solidification of solidarity for all the good times and bad times of the rest of our lives. It helped me become supremely confident that we were meant, more than ever, to be together—and that to me is a perfect foundation on which to bring a new life into the world.

TRY NUMBER TWO CAME WHEN HOPE HAD FOUND A permanent job over the summer and was feeling more confident and grounded in herself. Her sister was getting married the following year, in March, and we were trying to determine how many months she could be pregnant and still manage to be energized enough to be a good support for her sister during her wedding preparations and of course the big day.

You might think to yourself that the best time to try is to just try whenever you are ready. However, you might be surprised how much once-in-a-lifetime experiences play a part in your own life planning when it comes to this. It certainly took me a while to appreciate that. So with Hope in her job in July, the earliest month to try again was August, which of course still meant she would be two months off by the time March rolled in like a lion. And so off we went again, on the rollercoaster of cycle monitoring.

Wednesday, August 14th 2013 arrived. Up at 5:30 a.m. with a packed breakfast, a brewed coffee, and a kiss and off she went for an ultrasound and bloodwork. No $900 drug cost to delay this time. Day three, day five, day nine, day ten, eleven, thirteen... monitoring those hormone levels carefully.

Now, at this point, it might be worth mentioning that eight months earlier, Hope's second sister had announced that she was pregnant. We also had heard from our support group friends that a number of those couples had achieved pregnancy in two tries or under. I think there is likely a number of similar experiences for both partners—I am considering all manner of couples—as they move through the challenge of conceiving. However, I also imagine there is a *profound* difference between the person who will carry the child and have it grow inside them, and the partner who will witness and support the process.

I was genuinely ecstatic the moment anyone revealed their own amazing news to us. Of course, there were post-delighted thoughts lingering on the apparent ease with which others had achieved what we were working so hard to accomplish. What helped me was to stay real with how grateful I was—and am—and remind myself every single day of what I do have in my life to make that challenge feasible in the first place. I had—and have—a loving wonderful human being for a partner. I have a purposeful occupation to keep me engaged with my community. I live in a safe, warm, and comfortable house in a peaceful neighbour-hood. Both Hope and I have fantastic friendships in our lives to help process difficult feelings, both individually and as a couple. I have access to food that is safe and healthy and balanced. I have clean abundant drinking water. Yup, I am an incredibly fortunate human being.

Events happen when they happen, of course, but I did wonder what it would be like having a pregnant family member due in September a mere month after we had tried again. The mind tends to speculate and fantasize. Our child would have a cousin in the same year at school, but would be almost a year younger. And how lovely it would be to have that connection for both the children? I tried to not let my imagination get too carried away and not map out my potential child's entire life!

One thing I had learned from all the forms we had had to fill out and all choices we chose and decisions we had had to make thus far, was this: any child that resulted would be a rare privilege and it would be up to us to honour them as a new human being in their own right and guide and support them unconditionally. I knew that. The lengthy conversations we indulged each and every evening during these *trying* months often centred around how we would respond as a couple to discovering elements of our child—or children—that were not like us. How we would feel and think about it? How we would try to uncover ways to support it in a healthy and loving way regardless of our own preferences? I would try to search through my own process how to respond to these character traits. Tuesday August 27th rolled along and it was time to press the plunger on the syringe again. This time we were urged by the practitioner to do two units within twenty-four hours and so we spent double the dollars (around $5500) on this try. Thirteen days later, Hope started bleeding.

At first it was light, and so we deduced, in our clinging-onto-hope state, that it must be implantation bleeding. This is when the fertilized egg has reached the uterine lining and literally secures itself there. It is rather profound, the chemical reactions that occur that allow the attraction of nearby vessels to form and to connect or vascularise with the fertilized egg. And bingo we have a blood supply! The start of a nine-month gestation period.

At this point I had put all my energies into believing that it would happen this time, convincing my mind and spirit that it would happen. However, throughout the night her bleeding became heavier and heavier. She started to cry and I think at that point we already knew. So much for the Law of Attraction. However, it was a very emotionally confusing sensation because she had definitely felt profoundly different post-insemination. Hungry, fatigued, mood swings, physical pains. it is difficult to discern pregnancy symptoms from normal symptoms of pre-menstruation. hoping it was the former, they had been welcomed with open arms this time round!

With our two Dollar Store pregnancy tests—we had a spare just in case—it was time to confirm the status of the situation. And so, the morning of day fourteen, Hope went to pee on a stick. Sitting on the edge of the bath together, looking at the stick, it did not seem like a dramatic climax of the last number of weeks or months of building up to this point. It was a smack in our faces.

Negative.

Very cold. Very matter of fact. We knew it, yet seeing it helped the grieving, for me at least. There seemed to be some sense of control in preparing ourselves in advance before having it confirmed. Of course the final test was yet to come, and so we drove once more to the clinic to have one more blood test and one more phone call a couple of hours later to confirm no pregnancy.

"...so come in day three of your next cycle."

Six

NOW, I DO NOT KNOW ABOUT YOUR SITUATION, BUT with the thousands of dollars we had just spent and emotional rollercoaster we'd just ridden and the life disruption we'd just experienced, it was not going to be feasible for us to simply move on and start the monitoring with the intent to try again starting on day three of the next cycle (which is to say *two days later*). In cycle-monitoring terms, day 3 is considered the third day after you start bleeding again. Even if we were able to emotionally prepare ourselves and Hope were able to physically prepare *herself* to go through it all again, it was not realistic life-wise or financially. And so, we decided to give it a break.

If you are the kind of person who tends to set targets and limits, then it's easy in situations like this to get distraught. We'd told ourselves that we'd give it a couple of tries, and that if it didn't work, then we'd call it a day to focus on other goals. Well, here we were—unsuccessful after a couple of tries and reluctant to stick to our original plan. Like a self-imposed pressure.

It was hard to avoid feeling as though our physical bodies had let us down (mine at birth) and that we were being robbed of profound opportunity that occurs so naturally for others. Communication was so important here. One crook I always hold onto was how it is not anyone's *fault*, and that millions of people are in the same position. When we came out of our own individual story, and reflected on the countless other similar narratives, it helped us hold on to our blessings and maintain perspective. Remember, there is always, always, always something to be grateful for.

I had tried to save up all my vacation days and personal days at work for clinic times which could be unpredictable and often came up on short notice. So I had many left over and it was coming up to the last quarter of the year. And so I took a day off, plunked myself on a stool in a coffee shop, and wrote in my journal, trying to articulate my feelings about the whole experience. I wrote about how I understood that this had already done so much for our relationship—even my relationship with myself and life. I wrote about how I understood that I had worked hard for the things I had wanted in life and that all of those goals were really manifestations of love. That money was just a tool in my toolbox to enable and facilitate those manifestations of love—money was not love itself. And that at this point, if it was possible—and it would make us both happy and fulfil us—why *wouldn't* we give it another go?

Being able to come to this *on my own* was helpful. I felt as though I had gained some clarity. I sent a text to Hope whilst she was at work.

> don't worry, I have a plan and everything
> will be OK

She reminded me later about this message and how much hope it brought to her. When I saw her at the end of the day and told her how I felt we ought to keep planning and trying, she was filled with relief and hope again. Funny how it is not the achievement of the goal that brings these memories to fruition, but the will and perseverance itself. I am still learning this in many aspects of my life.

The next month, my first niece was born. It was rather amazing to be on the periphery of the couple going through the motions of birth. Truth be told, many of our friends and acquaintances had had babies in the last couple of years—most without the need of any sort of medical intervention. There was a bittersweet sort of wonder to that.

We were privileged to be able to visit our niece in hospital the same day. From the intermittent phone calls from the doula throughout the night, to hearing the announcement of her birth, right up to seeing her on the same day she entered the world was a profound honour for me.

We had not been explicit with Hope's extended family about our issues around infertility. And though it is natural for people to form assumptions about all sorts of things—everyone does, myself included—it is odd that, when it comes to trying to get pregnant, so few people stop and wonder if there are fertility issues at play.

Even oblique hints like "yes we're trying, but it's taking a while" or "it's not as easy as we thought" don't necessarily point folks in the right direction.

> "Ah well, it's fun to try, right?" Wink.

> "Heck, enjoy the process." Shoulder slap. "It might take a few months before it works."

> "Just relax, and it will happen when it happens..."

Even folks who did know the big picture (medically) didn't seem to grasp what we were going through.

"Just try again. No biggie."

It felt pretty socially isolating even though I knew folks were trying to be encouraging. Really the only other person who seemed to appreciate what we were going through was Hope. I took the positive energy and tried to forget the unintended ignorance. Some people discount intention when staked up against results, but not me. If something is well intended, I will take those positive intentions even if the gesture itself was ill-conceived or downright dumb. Which isn't to say that I always accepted boneheaded comments with grace and poise—I didn't—only to say that I would always take what I could in the way of positive energy from folks willing to offer it.

It's important to remember that all of us go through so much in our lives, sometimes these are short-term lessons, sometimes long-term, and that no one has a monopoly on wisdom. We can all learn from each one another. For me, the bottom line is that learning is only effective and worth anything if it is done with loving kindness. If an interaction brings no learning for me but brings with it an intention of love, I'll take the intention.

WE WERE SO DAMN EXHAUSTED FROM DRIVING TO and from the clinic all the time for invasive procedures that afterwards we just wanted quiet sleep time. I got quite run down a number of times because of the toll of the whole process and the stress it induced. Trying again involved planning our entire life schedule around it for months and assigning at least $3500 to pay for the process which involved sacrifices and prioritizing other projects.

As a couple we had already been through a lot of reflection together to understand and know in our hearts that (a) it was not our fault (b) that we could only control the facilitation of chances and that the rest was up to the universe, and (c) we were simply going to have to keep trying—although it was very kind of folks to remind us!!

AUTUMN IS MY FAVOURITE SEASON, AND LIVING IN Canada, the autumn colours are spectacular. It is a beautiful display of the lifecycle of nature all around us and evokes, in me, a sense of a new beginning. How apt that was for my soul that year.

In the October of 2013, we decided to take a few months' break and give ourselves a bit of a vacation, and Cuba was the location.

I had not seen my mother for over a year, not since the wedding, and since October was right after her birthday month, we brought her to Cuba to meet up with us. We talked, we reflected, we walked along the beach, we read a lot of books, and it calmed my spirit down. One recurring thought I had was that I wished, with all my heart, for my mother to meet my child. I felt that each interaction they would be able to have would mean that her spirit would live on in my child once she was no longer walking the Earth. That became a very strong wish for me. It occurred to me that nature and nurture were the two arenas influencing development and that we had carefully selected the nature part that was ours to select, and that nurture would be the rest of the child's influence. My mother shared with me a lot of her life wisdom, and that afforded me a great deal of perspective, and I recognized how lucky I was to have the family I had.

Flying back to Canada, we discussed when out next *try* would be. The money was there because we had gotten so used to saving that it really was not too much of a problem to maintain the life adjustments mentioned earlier! We decided it would be December since we were returning at the end of October and had missed the cycle monitoring for November.

That month I was visited by a thought that had popped into my head many times before.

I wonder who the person from this month's egg would have been...

Seven

DECEMBER ROLLED AROUND RATHER QUICKLY, AND it was time to buy some more units of sperm so they could be shipped in time for the insemination day. We went back online. It had been a while since we had done this, just under a year in fact. We realized that, at this point, we were free to review our choice and essentially start all over again. We browsed through the folks who met the criteria we had decided upon and found the original donor still came up. We reviewed his profile and lo and behold he had gotten divorced. Obviously pretty much everything else had stayed the same. And as ridiculous as it sounds, for it would not be making a difference to the sperm whatsoever, that was enough to make us change our minds and land on a different donor altogether! There is nothing wrong with divorce, and perhaps that was the best and most mature decision for that person—I think it was more a case of we were in a different place, and we were looking for another "change" to permit our decision to change.

The second donor was from a whittled list of about three. We had read their essays and searched for character traits that were not tangible although we had kept the filters of similar physical traits. This time, we found someone who seemed to have not been on the list before, and he was even a similar age to me (most donors were in their twenties). This person looked a little bit like me in some of his photos, and it had shown that his donations had been successful in helping a few couples conceive. It eventually came down to him and one other donor. The ultimate reason for picking this one was because we had determined, based on our own arbitrary criteria, that the donor's skillset would balance out Hope's skillset nicely. Whether any of these skills were actually innate or not would not be knowable, but just in case, we went with it nonetheless.

This time we were going to order and use, in the same cycle, two units from this donor. The first time we had ordered two units as well, however, the nurse recommended, when it came to it, that we just use one unit—we used the second unit for our second attempt.

We were hopeful, again, that this would boost our chances, and there was a renewed energy with the process. We also decided that we would, as Hope put it, have her pipes cleaned—which is to say we would invest in a sonohysterogram! Apparently that can sometimes increase the chances. By this point—because of the almost $10,000 worth of investments we had made—we wanted to make absolutely sure there was nothing that was obstructing or making it more difficult for us to conceive. We had consulted the doctor who warned us that though it was a free procedure (at least in Canada) it was a painful one, and to take some Tylenol in preparation. The timing of the test was not great-they only did this procedure every Tuesday and Wednesday within an hour time slot. Person-centred the system is not, in case you hadn't figured that out by now.

The doctor wasn't kidding about the sonohysterogram. Even with the Tylenol it was painful, and though of the two of us Hope got the short end of the stick again, it's hard watching the one you love in pain. You need to remind yourself to simply be present for your partner and focus on everything you have to be thankful for. By the time it was done we had something else to be thankful for. If showed no blockages or obstructions whatsoever.

I had not taken a lot of vacation all year because I wanted to support Hope on clinic days, and doing so would require me to be away from work, and so I held onto them—not that I'd had to use one for insemination day yet (we delayed until the weekend the first time and I was between jobs the second time). It was the same old routine as before. Back and forth to the clinic we went, with blood tests and ultrasounds. However, this time, because the clinic had come to know her cycle quite well, the doctor told us to not bother coming in to see how big the follicle had grown and how much her estrodiol levels had risen until day thirteen, estradiol being an estrogen sex hormone produced in the ovaries. We went back on day fourteen, being told the inseminations might be Thursday and Friday—to *sandwich* the actual moment of ovulation. We went back on day fifteen and were told maybe Friday and Saturday. On day sixteen we were told probably Saturday and Sunday. So, it turned out once again we were expecting insemination on a weekend! Convenient, don't you think?

Saturday came and in we went. However, once there we were told *definitely* Sunday and Monday. And so it went that I finally got to use one of my floater days! If you can negotiate a floater day with your work in your contract it is *very* useful. And so, on the Sunday, we went in, filled out the familiar consent form—*I will not sue you if this does not work or if this child has unforeseen issues.* Seriously, the world has come to that. Do folks without fertility issues sue God if that happens without clinical intervention? Finally, of course, the consent for the sperm to be thawed was paw printed too. It was a very quiet day this time. December 15,

2013, with not many folks around. We had again tried to gauge the parking, and this time paid the four bucks for all-day parking we'd discovered across the street. Oh yes, we were willing to splash out for this entire experience!

The previous two times we had been asked to wait for several hours until being called in ready for thawed sperm to be inseminated. However, this time we were told to come back at 9:30 after signing off the forms at 8:30, and when we did wander back to the clinic, they told us they'd been ready for a while. Keep smiling in these moments or else you will go insane!

We were ushered into the insemination room and prepared ourselves—we knew the drill. Initially the receptionist mentioned that the doctor would be in shortly, but we were not taking any more crap and spoke up rather abruptly to say we had specifically requested a particular provider and were aware they were available. It can be quite liberating to advocate for yourself, and in this case the receptionist was, well, receptive! There was a CD player in the room, and I proceeded to press play and turn up the volume to music that was Zen-like in sound, and it really helped relax us and feel at peace with the situation. *Always* a good idea when an invasive procedure is around the corner to bring whatever helps you:, an iPod, photos, anything.

A few minutes later the nurse came in with the vial and warmed up the speculum, and as I held Hope's hand and sang to her to distract her, the nurse prepared the syringe and held it ready for me to push the swimmers in—and so I did. Fifteen minutes later, we were ready to leave. It takes about ten seconds to push the syringe of an insemination procedure, and then it is pretty much done. We were due to go to a party in the afternoon and debated about staying out. That lasted a few milliseconds before we decided it would be best to go home first and rest up since we were both exhausted from the early mornings and emotionally heightened state.

THE NEXT DAY STARTED WITH ANOTHER EARLY morning and another trip to the clinic for the *second* insemination to up the odds. It had snowed heavily the night before, so I wanted to make absolutely sure we would get there in time and safely. The pressure is really on when the window is twelve to twenty-four hours for that egg, although it is up to seventy-two hours for the sperm to hang around inside!

This time the clinic was a lot busier, and we did not park across the street but in a supermarket car park, presuming it would be a similar situation—we will never learn about the blasted parking?! Heads up, if you are going to spend this much money trying to have a baby, allow yourself the luxury of not having to worry about parking. Heck we had spent near to $5,000 and more on this process this time round, what the heck is an extra few bucks? Blame it on the long-term thrift required to afford this whole process in the first place! You'll know what I am talking about if this is where you are at. The supermarket was a ten-minute walk away from the clinic, and so we had a quick breakfast of cold meat and bagels and strolled back down the hill to be ready for the *back-up shot*.

We were eventually called in around 10:30.

Now, when you are ready to be inseminated, the protocol is that they show the lab results of the sperm to show you how motile the sperm are and how many of them there are—these are approximate numbers, of course. All three previous units had shown results of between eight and eleven million sperm and motility of between two and four (on a scale of zero to four). They also could show you what percentage of the thawed sperm were active—the previous shots all fell between the forty to fifty-five percent range. However, this unit was ninety-five percent active at a motility of three to four and the count was seventeen million sperm strong!

That is when I felt that this is going to be a bloody good shot! Once again we asked for our preferred provider who was incredibly gentle and calm and respectful and talked us through the whole process. In this business, bedside manner means everything to the patient—providers take note!

Holding Hope's hand once more, and praying for and with her, the nurse set up the speculum and syringe, inviting me to push. This time I pushed slightly faster to give the swimmers that extra boost. The nurse had looked at us and mentioned that ovulation was *definitely* occurring right now. At that point, I *knew* we could not have done anything better, timed it any better, or worked any harder to make this happen. And now it was up to nature, God, the universe—the myriad magical factors all beyond our control.

All we had left to do was to wait.

THIS WAS THE CHRISTMAS SEASON AND RELATIVELY a good time to be waiting given all the built-in distractions of the holidays. In 2013, this included an eleven-day power outage in Toronto and the Greater Toronto Area due to a freak ice storm that downed thousands of power lines and trees. Gratefully we were only affected for three and a half days—although at minus twenty-five degrees Celsius it felt darn longer than that! My in-laws let us sleep in their home, which had not been affected by the outage, and we kept shuttling back and forth to our house to make sure no pipes had burst and all the other potential delights one might encounter in such a time.

We spent Christmas with my in-laws at a farmhouse my sister-in-law and her fiancé had recently bought. It was a very romantic day, and of course, we got to see our lovely niece. She was truly amazing to see, so engaging at the tender age of three months. I could not keep my mind from wandering and casting glances at Hope's tummy. I was very glad for the distractions of other people's lives over that period. Neither of us had taken any holidays over this period. Subconsciously, I suspect we wanted work as an additional distraction while waiting for the dreaded two weeks to pass.

By the second half of the second week, we were getting antsy to test. It is actually possible to detect a positive pregnancy with certain tests that are designed for early responses to hCG, or human Chorionic Gonadotrophin hormone, which is essentially is considered the *pregnancy hormone*. And naturally we were watching acutely for signs and symptoms and immediately went to the internet with anything we detected. It was a pointless compulsion, and we knew it, but what else were we going to do?! We'd been cautioned by folks told to not invest our time in Google, that we'd drive ourselves nuts, but who is *not* going to research the symptoms they experience? Who, from the pool of people determined to at least try to conceive, is not going to try to empower themselves somehow, some way, no matter how under-read someone else thinks they are? I ask you. I think the best advice might sound something like this:

> Go do whatever it is you have to do to feel
> in control and manage the emotional roll-
> ercoaster you are experiencing. If you feel

*compelled to go to the internet, go for it. But
don't just look at Google. Look at scholarly
articles, look at books, talk to people, gather as
much information as you can both anecdotal
and experiential because I am just one provider, and I am a human being. I was schooled
one specific way, but of course there are
others. I am delighted to be a part of your team
to try and will try my best to make this miracle
happen. And I will see you in two weeks.*

Boxing day fell on a Thursday, and though our clinic appointment was scheduled for Monday December 30, we cracked and
decided that we were going to test. We are not big shoppers and
so the Boxing Day crowds didn't distract us! And so although we
knew it would likely turn out negative because it was too soon, we
got a pee stick.

Of course, it turned out negative.

Yet, strangely, this gave us peace, and we were able to let it go
another day. On Friday we were working again, which made things
easier, but then on Saturday, we were going out of our minds
whether to test or not. It is a real mind fuck when you know that
you're in the grips of an irrational compulsion but there is nothing
you can do about it. In the end we decided that we weren't
hurting anyone or jeopardizing anything so why not just succumb
and scratch the itch. We decided we'd would get an early response
test from Walmart.

I was feeling anxious at this point. I just kept telling Hope that
whatever happens it would all work out for the best and that we
were going to have a family no matter what the result. And of
course, that was true for we already were a family.

Emotions had been running high all day, and were feeling increasingly confused as there are several symptoms that are signs of pregnancy but also signs of imminent menstruation. Hope did mention that she did feel a bit different this time. This I must admit got me excited, but I could not allow myself to get too excited. At the same time, I didn't want to hedge my hopes just to protect myself from disappointment. I didn't know how to feel. Like I said, a mind fuck.

Please God. Please God. Please God...

We got in the car. We drove to the Walmart. We got out of the car. We went into Walmart. We went to the section for early response pregnancy test kits. We looked at the early response pregnancy test kits. We compared prices. We looked at each other.

We decided to not get one.

We left Walmart, got back in the car, and drove home.

These kind of behaviours of acting out the entire sequence of events and not actually getting to the final stage seemed to be very helpful in managing the anxiety. Sometimes, during those final few days of our two-week wait, it really came down to how we were going to get through the next half hour let alone an entire night. This I am told is how hope works in the human brain, rationalizing an optimism bias and visualizing the future you would like to participate in: how's that for clinical?

Sunday. Let's just say Sunday was a train wreck. We took a test and it was negative—this was definitely past the day it would show. Later we took *another* test... and got another negative. Needless to say, the hope poured out of us like sand out of a smashed hourglass.

Hope was in mourning. Even as I comforted her, I told myself that it was not over and that we could try again. We didn't even bother getting a blood test—the next day her body told us it was over.

Eight

MY MUM HAD COME TO STAY WITH US FROM THE UK, and staying positive during this grieving process was obviously painfully difficult, but I was very open with my mum, and she was very supportive and understanding as always. I sometimes worried about myself as I never cried at any of these failed attempts for pregnancy. I just accepted them each time. I seemed to find a safe space in being philosophical about it all—probably easier for me to do since I was not the one going through the physical aspect of the trying process. Obviously I was incredibly frustrated, and at times infuriated.

Thank God for distractions.

Christmas had come and gone, an ice storm had cut the power off for days, and of course we had Mum with us. Seeing the opportunities in the difficulties is a practice: this time that practice included a trip to see Niagara Falls frozen by a freak polar vortex. It lasted for about forty-eight hours, and during this rare occurrence, I was able to drive my mum and myself there to see it. That was something quite amazing and a welcome relief to see nature create something beautiful whilst also so fleeting. It reminded me of the fleetingness of pregnancy tries. It comes, it happens, and when it fails, it's gone. The frozen falls were something to witness, and they reminded me of the profound strength of spirit of folks involved in this journey in my life from which I gained courage.

My mum and I had travelled a lot together in our lives, and I'm sure I inherited my restless soul from her. In fact, everything good about my foundations came from her, and set the stage for being able to fight for everything good about my wonderful relationship with Hope. These were the two people to whom I held myself accountable. If either of them questioned anything I thought or did, I would give it more thought and reflection. Otherwise I trusted myself.

Life of course never ceases for anyone or anything, and it was odd for me to see a co-worker in the office suddenly balloon up seemingly overnight, and shortly thereafter announce that she was three months pregnant. I was immediately happy for her, and it was a welcome, hopeful sight to see it happen physically for someone else. I congratulated her and wished her and her partner all the best for the future. In the meantime, my capacity to say *yes* to any work that was headed my way was getting tanked. I could see that what I had been doing was trying to drown myself in my work to keep myself as busy as possible, and when that happens, it is amazing how much work of little or no consequence there is to do! It was not until I was doing up to seventy hours a week that I could see that it was not sustainable, or smart.

If there is something I have learned in the last ten years or so, it's that I need to be more direct and take personal responsibility for my well-being. I had noticed that my reasoning up to that point was that I would keep working insane hours until I had children and then I would pull back. Thankfully, I had a partner who was able to give me insight into what a ridiculous and self-harming approach this was. Why wait until then? Good question. By the time that happened the bar would have already been set and pulling back would be hard to impossible to do. Boundaries would need to be set now and relationships recalibrated to a healthier place.

The only effective way I could think of was pulling out of my calendar, line by line, all the pieces I had been doing, and giving an accurate accounting of them to my superiors. It was certainly an eye-opener. It was enough for me to literally say "no" to new work and to be clear in my boundaries around work. The fear I'd instilled in myself about the need for insane work hours was unfounded, and I saw that now. I had solid rational boundaries, and that boosted my confidence to pursue long-term sustainable balance so that I could meaningfully channel my energy.

It's too easy to let something like what Hope and I were pursuing serve as a blank check for unsustainable decision making. If we were hoping to have a child, didn't it make more sense that we were adding that new life to lives already in balance?

Nine

THE NEW YEAR FELT FRESH AND MORE FOCUSED than years gone by. My mum was still visiting us when Hope and I wrote down our goals and hopes for 2014 and tallied what we saw as our accomplishments of 2013. We read them to each other like testimonies of our wills to persevere and to honour the struggles we had been through.

The first item on my list of goals was to try again for a baby. At this point it just seemed natural. That night Hope and I sat in bed and discussed it. It was first on her list too. I guess we just knew at that we had to keep going. Our understanding was that, on average, folks who tried to conceive through intra-uterine insemination could expect it to take between four and six tries—after which other medical interventions might be considered.

We gave ourselves a break for January and actually considered IVF (in vitro fertilization)... for about five nanoseconds. For Hope and I, the thought of putting her body through so much, not to mention the crippling financial costs of up to $20,000 per try and the fact that those costs bought you no guarantees, meant that IVF was a no go for us. For Hope this meant going through the rigours of IUI, which involved regular invasive ultrasounds and needle pricks and catheters and syringes and sonohysterograms.

And so, in February of 2014, the cycle monitoring started up all over again. At this point, it had just become a routine part of our lives to get up early and see her off in the dark so that she could drive to the clinic alone, have these procedures done, and get on with the rest of our day. I knew that I was doing everything I could do within my control and that life was now becoming less focused on whether or not it would work and more about incorporating these routine practices into our lives for the foreseeable future.

This was our fourth time. We had been attending this clinic for a year, and in that time, the clinic had grown and had received their own addition to their team family. A new doctor was on the books, and we had an appointment with this newbie. This doctor advised us that one try was enough per insemination, and that is when we had to dig a little deeper to understand that there were varying perspectives between doctors as to whether one or two units was best. Bear in mind that the difference between one and two inseminations is potentially thousands of dollars. More on this particular topic later, but the larger lesson here is not to take anything *one* doctor says as gospel truth. When differences of opinion exist within a single fertility clinic, you begin to realize the importance of doing your own research and pursuing second opinions.

In discussing how best to up the odds of our next attempt, the drug Clomid came up as an option worth consideration. Clomid is an ovulation induction drug that is used to increase the number of active follicles in a given cycle and thus increase the potential number of eggs. Now, here's the thing: the effects of Clomid are unique to each person and careful monitoring is done to ensure that would-be parents are aware of how many potential pregnancies might occur.

What is happening with Clomid, as one doctor put it, is that you are increasing the number of targets the sperm can fertilize and, therefore, increasing the chances of a pregnancy. Obviously you are also increasing the chances of *multiple* fertilizations in one cycle. For some people their body responds to Clomid by producing two eggs instead of one, for others it can be up to five eggs—*or more*. So although the chance is a small, it is *possible* that, on Clomid, you could end up with five embryos implanted!

This was a serious consideration. Maybe you are okay with having five children you couldn't hope to support—to each their own—for me and Hope it was important to ensure could that we could support a child (or children) and properly provide for them. Quality of life was a more important consideration than mere quantity of life.

During that week of early morning cycle monitoring, we saw different doctors. This is when it got really interesting, for different doctors were offering conflicting information. One doctor was upset to hear that another doctor had told us two inseminations per cycle make no difference, for there had been a study to prove that two does make a difference. However, a third doctor told us that more and more studies were showing that two makes no difference and advised us to just use one. There was also a list forthcoming from each camp as to all the reasons they were likely right—they had been practicing longer; they sat on certain boards and committees; the relative credentials of the various studies, etc.

This was a moment I truly recall being incredibly proud of Hope. She had been persistent in her questioning of the facts and enquiring and was not intimidated-she wanted to stay until she got these answers. If we learned anything from this experience it was to ask questions and keep asking until you are satisfied.

We ordered two more units of sperm while all of this was going on to ensure that the units arrived in time. We eventually settled into the single insemination camp, however; and it was reassuring—even if just from a financial perspective—to reflect that two out of the three times we had tried so far, we had just used one insemination. As for the double inseminations on the last try, well, it was good if only to shake things up and try something different.

Einstein suggested that the best definition of insanity is doing the same thing over and over again and expecting a different result. But this didn't quite fit the true definition of insanity because of course, at three attempts, we were still within the anecdotal odds for success, and persistence is not the same as insanity because, each time you try, you are growing stronger or learning something new. Insanity is when there is nothing to learn (or, worse, when there *is* and you refuse to learn it) and all odds point to their there being a problem.

We were ready to move forward with a single insemination attempt. With the two units we had just purchased, if the next attempt didn't work the second unit could be for the *following* attempt. We also concluded that if this attempt was unsuccessful that we would start on the Clomid pills for the following cycle. It was good to know that we already had a plan in place in the event of a fourth unsuccessful attempt. I think it helped relieve the pressure a bit knowing that we weren't putting all of our eggs in one basket (so to speak).

THIS TIME AROUND, THE MONITORING INDICATED that insemination day was earlier than expected (which is why they monitor these things). Once again, it was a Saturday, which makes it a lot easier to arrange when you work Monday to Friday! We had this process down to a fine art: park the car at the subway station for $4 all day; get the ultrasound done, which showed that ovulation was imminent (i.e. that day most likely); and arrange to inseminate a little bit early—we were told that sperm, including frozen sperm, can live inside the body post-thawing for up to five days. So the consent was signed for thawing, and off we went for coffee (well coffee for me and herbal tea for her) and a breakfast sandwich at a local coffee shop. Yes, we spoiled ourselves by *splitting* a breakfast sandwich. Then it was back to the clinic about an hour later.

We waited in the room for the doctor who had seen us for most of this cycle time to come and do the insemination. When the doctor arrived we were told that the unit details were also good, at fourteen million sperm in the sample, with high motility and percent viable. We were far less anxious and eager to try something different, so we asked the doctor to push the plunger while I held my darling's hand. The doctor agreed and mentioned that there was, in fact, an optimal speed at which to plunge it without "scaring" the sperm. News to us. While the doctor did the deed, I looked into Hope's eyes and told her how much I loved her.

It may sound strange to you, but afterwards I wanted to keep the vial. I had this idea in my head that, if I'd been conceived this way, it would be so awesome to one day hold the vial that had held the sperm that made me! So I took it with me. If you are symbolic like this, just speak up.

Fifteen minutes later, we were leaving the room, filled with hope and all the positive feelings we could possible muster.

Because it was a Saturday, we went back home and slept. We were, as always, pretty exhausted from the whole thing—the early mornings, the preliminary procedures and paperwork, the waiting, the anticipation, the emotions. It is a lot to process.

That evening we went out to a belated Lunar New Year's party. As usual, no alcohol or "wrong foods for pregnancy" such as raw fish. We had already prepared pineapple core and other *interesting* foods that are apparently good for increasing the odds. Unless it's a natural food product, I personally would not worry too much about this. That being said when it comes to supporting one's partner, I say let them do what they need to do!

However, you don't have to eat it!

Just as I drank the alcohol that she didn't have to drink. Fair's fair after all. This party, we knew, would be the start of another long two weeks of waiting.

Ten

THE TIME TO TEST CAME, AND THE ELUSIVE PEE-
stick second line we prayed for never came. Attempt number four
had failed.

I won't sugar-coat things. It was incredibly depressing. It was a
Sunday morning, and at that moment, the house felt as quiet as a
tomb. Then suddenly the atmosphere switched from powerless-
ness to determination, and we jumped into the car to go to the
clinic and get ourselves some Clomid. We were not ready to give
up. We were now ready for the next step of treatment.

Clomid is a drug you take in pill form. Because everyone reacts
differently to it, we started on the smallest recommended dose,
50mg. Here's how Here's Clomid works: in the normal course of
events, what triggers the ovaries to produce a follicle is a hormone
released by the pituitary gland—known simply enough as follicle
stimulating hormone or FSH. The new follicle (or rather the egg
inside it) emits oestrogen. The extra oestrogen in the blood, gets
back to the pituitary gland, located at the base of the brain, and
attaches itself to oestrogen receptors there. When those receptors are thus triggered, the pituitary gland duly slows down and
stops releasing FSH. That ensures that, most of the time, only one
follicle, and therefore one egg, becomes matured per menstrual

cycle. However, Clomid attaches itself to oestrogen receptors on the pituitary gland and, by doing so, blocks the oestrogen in the blood from properly activating the receptors thus preventing the pituitary gland from shutting down FSH production. Therefore, the FSH levels remain high and the ovaries to continue to grow follicles.

The whole point of this process, of course, is to end up with more targets for the sperm to hit, thus increasing the odds of conception. But that's not all. Furthermore, Clomid helps increase the chance of viability of the egg (or eggs) being released. Without Clomid, there is higher chance that the egg (or eggs) released from the follicles are not quite mature enough to be viable. Of course there is absolutely no way of knowing when this occurs.

We knew all of this already, which is why, when we hopped in the car that Sunday, we were determined to advocate hard for Clomid. I was gearing up for a bit of a fight because, although we'd heard about the clinic's so-called stepped approach to fertility support *many times* over the past year, it was suggested to us the previous week that Clomid was going to require a separate consultation appointment. This would have to be booked, would no doubt occur in the middle of the week, would require both of us to coordinate time off, and would not afford us any new information. We did not want to miss a cycle just to hear all this again.

I mean, honestly, what was there to discuss? We had already spent a year talking about it. It was dead simple. A stepped approach to fertility support. Yes, we got it (we even agreed with it). We'd now had four unsuccessful IUI attempts. The next step was Clomid at the smallest dose. We did not want to waste time waiting for a consultation to tell us what we already knew. We needed to keep going; no more breaks. Time was ticking away. We already had the next batch of sperm on ice, and Hope's next cycle was cued up.

The other issue that concerned me was that, although we'd been assigned a designated doctor, because the clinic had a rotating schedule, when you dropped in, you got whomever was in the clinic at the time. In other words, we weren't sure who we were going to end up seeing. Though I had psyched myself up to fight, as we drove I became less and less confident that we were going to walk out of there with Clomid and didn't want to face a second disappointment (even if only in the form of a delay) that day. At one point I even asked if we should turn back and leave it a month.

No dice. Hope was adamant we should try, and so we kept driving. That's the thing about being in a partnership, you can each act as cheerleader for each other when spirits sink or confidence falters.

We arrived, and discovered a newer doctor was in the house. We articulated the approach we were determined to take—this included bombarding the doctor with facts we already knew about Clomid, how long we'd been trying, our need to switch designated doctors, and the reasons why it was not fair to force us to wait and miss a cycle. We made it clear that, while we understood the doctor's need to act ethically and appropriately, it was important that our case be considered reasonably on its own merits.

We got *everything* out of our system before the doctor responded.

"Okay well that's a lot to address. Let's start with the changing of your designated doctor. That's not our policy here so—"

"So I guess the only way for us to change doctors then is to go to another clinic," Hope said, thinking that they wouldn't want to lose our business.

The doctor took a deep breath and offered a tired smile.

She said something to the effect of "I was *about* to say that that's not our policy here, but it's the doctor's responsibility to keep you happy, so please just ensure that the doctor you've been assigned is aware of your issues so she can work them out."

Our main problem with the doctor we'd been assigned was that she was the only one pressing for a double insemination (based on the strength of one study) and we had already changed camps on that issue. She also struck us as slightly inflexible and intransigent in her beliefs. She just wasn't a good fit. I was about to go into the ethics of not being able to change doctors and the role of stress and a good fit between doctor and patient when on-duty doc spoke up again.

"All that being said, I would be happy to prescribe you Clomid today."

Yes, I thought, *well done team!*

The doctor assured us that it was clear we had had enough consultation on this stuff already, which goes to show that strong lucid self-advocacy is important and can be effective. Know what you're talking about and present a solid argument.

That day we ended up doing another unexpected ultrasound and blood test before starting the Clomid the next day. The side effects were headaches, tiredness and bloating, but they were all manageable—particularly for me because I wasn't experiencing them! My role was to be as supportive and as patient as possible.

Hope was to take the Clomid for five days, and a few days after her last pill, we went in to have an ultrasound and discovered that her body had responded to the treatment by growing two eggs instead of one.

Great! If we ended up with two babies, then we would go through the stages all at once with both of them.

Insemination was scheduled a few days later.

Eleven

WE LUCKED OUT AGAIN, FOR THE TIMING MEANT that insemination day landed *once more* on a weekend. We knew going into the procedure that our odds had shot up from eight percent to a twenty-five percent chance of pregnancy on Clomid—I had asked for the stats from our clinic and this is what we were shown. Now although that was still only a one in four chance, it was more than three times the odds of previous attempts, based on a certain body of research, and that felt empowering and gave us hope. One in four is a significant chance. And we were praying and hoping that this would be it.

However, the initial news was less than ideal. After washing the sperm we had just unfrozen, the count was low. At seven million that was lower than the all the others—although the motility was very good. I tried to keep things positive, suggesting it was quality not quantity, and pointing out that we had doubled the targets and that we only needed that one of those seven million to make it.

In the back of my mind, however, I was less positive.

You've gotta be kidding me.

Alas, I had to relinquish again yet another step that was out of my control. There was simply nothing I could do about what the count and motility was going to end up being. That is simply par for the course.

We started the insemination process, and for some reason, this time, Hope could not relax—which is actually important. It was never a pleasant experience, of course, speculums and syringes being what they are. It's possible that the past attempts plus the added odds from the Clomid this time combined to ratchet up the pressure. Of course the early morning didn't help either, and the nerves the night before... and as time passed, it started to get more distressing, until eventually the nurse explained that she would need to get the doctor to come in to help her with this procedure.

A word of advice here, when it comes to relaxation, bring whatever works to the table. Chocolate, music, soothing words, hair stroking. And do a lot of research on muscle and ligament connections in the groin area of the potential birth parent. If she can relax certain parts of her body all the muscles connected will follow and allow the procedure to occur. The best I can describe it is focusing on the bum muscles, the ones that you clench to make your arse look well worked out, and then breathing into relaxing them. Hey, it worked for us.

With the syringe pressed and the swimmers—all seven million of them—sent on their merry way, the doctor suggested we consider progesterone supplements. Not that Hope's progesterone levels were an issue, conception-wise, but it has been shown to be helpful for folks in general to prevent potential miscarriages should one become pregnant. At this point we agreed to anything that might help.

THE TWO WEEKS OF WAITING IT WAS.

We'd managed one small spiritual victory this time by resisting the urge to test early. However, when it *was* time to test, the elusive second line on the pee stick, once again, did not appear.

This time it was especially hard to hear the negative result because we had tried something different and been so diligent taking these extra medicinal supports. Of course, a one in four chance of success means a three in four chance of failure. Even so, in the back of my mind, I was starting to despair that maybe it was never going to happen. I could tell Hope was feeling that way too. We reminded each other that it had only been five times and *not* out of the ordinary. I reflected that maybe it had not worked because of exhaustion, and of course the procedure had not gone well that time—plus of course the sperm count was lower.

There is so much that is out of your control. It can drive you crazy if you let it.

Hell, for that matter, it could be that the biochemistry of this particular donor was simply not a viable match for Hope's. This was a maddening little wrinkle we'd been informed of early on in the process, one that could not be tested for. What is one supposed to do with that piece of information?

Anyway, we left ourselves very little time to grieve, and focussed instead on our next move. Either we could try Clomid again or go onto something more aggressive. We were told about the side effects of the next step which was an injectable drug that blocks the same pituitary gland receptors as Clomid, but is shown to be more aggressive. A less aggressive alternative was to simply up the dose of Clomid.

Either way, the goal seemed to be increase the number of eggs, for there was no arguing with the math of more eggs. The nurse had advised just going straight onto the more aggressive inject-able menupur, and so that is what we decided.

We picked them up from the doctor who showed Hope how to self-inject. As an aside, I have to do self-injections of testosterone every few weeks to manage my own medical condition, so I knew that I could, in fact, help out here a little bit with administering them. However, Hope managed to do it solo, with just me being present, and outdid me by far when I first had to learn my own self-injection regimen! So my role I guess was to cheerlead as much as possible.

I was grateful that my work's benefits package covered a limited amount of fertility drugs. It didn't cover the procedures them-selves or other pieces of the puzzle that cost a small fortune, but the drug coverage was better than nothing.

As with the Clomid, the injectables were to be administered for five days, then we were to go back in and monitor the egg and fol-licle development and potentially take them for *another* five days then review. In the meantime, we needed to order new sperm, and the decision needed to be made whether to stick with the same donor that had produced such a wide variety of counts and motility. And the decision was a new contestant-it made sense to change up every variable at this point.

We had also been busy getting on with day-to-day life. Two days after we found out about the failure of the Clomid attempt, my mother had come over to Canada—this was a few days before we started on the injectables. All of which is to say it was an incred-ibly busy and stressful period. My mum staying was a welcome support and distraction in the evenings for me, for it meant I did not have to think too much about it when I did not have to.

Our teamwork on our mission had isolated us a bit. I think that's probably pretty normal as it required a lot of time, money and attention to pursue—and at the same time it's an incredibly personal affair. If you are not careful it can really take a toll on your health, both physically and mentally. We forced ourselves to get to bed as early as possible, which seemed to help. I had been incredibly ill the last month with four separate infections, from angular cheilitis to strep throat to bronchitis to tooth infections involving the removal of two wisdom teeth. And it was this experience that had forced me to take a step back and re-evaluate how much unnecessary energy I had been expending at work. I realized that I had thrown myself into my job to help me cope with feeling not in control and being the support partner, watching someone I love going through all the physical side of this journey.

THE COURSE OF INJECTABLES RAN FOR FIVE DAYS. Then it was back to the clinic for the monitoring of initial results-two initial eggs. The next ten days required 6 a.m. trips to the clinic for injections of a daily dose of Bravelle , an additional injectable, to encourage maturity of eggs—but not too many. We chose for the clinic to administer where we could although we learned along the way to do it ourselves-a helpful skill to have on this journey. As exhausting as that was for us, we were accepting of the situation and took things one day at a time. There were detailed daily reports which meant something to the doctors but very little to us. We just did what we were told.

This time, when it finally came to the actual insemination, we were encouraged to do a "trigger" shot of manufactured Human chorionic gonadotropin, to stimulate ovulation, the day before to ensure ovulation would occur within a timed 36-hour window.

This helps improve the timing of things and increases the chance of conception

I have to tell you, the instructions for the trigger shot were not exactly clear and concise. The message left by the clinic was to take the shot at 2 p.m. which of course we didn't get to hear until closer to 7 p.m. once we were home from work. To top it off, the syringe of this trigger shot did not seem to be working, for the instructions had failed to explain the need to twist and pull back on the syringe first *before* injecting, so that took a bit of patience and grace under pressure.

Eventually we got it in, and the next day was the insemination. It had to be early as we both needed to run off afterwards to our respective employers. We were told that Hope's body had shown signs of maturing three eggs in total. That was not much considering what an aggressive regimen she had just endured. And although we had gone through this a few times before we were no less tense than before-the future of our family were depending on the outcome. I was actually more anxious this time to the point that I wanted the practitioner to push the plunger and I didn't keep the vial. I played games in my head that all these different choices over things I had a choice over would influence the outcome.

IN THE FERTILITY WORLD, WHAT CAME NEXT IS known rather pedantically as "the two week wait." After that the blood test at the clinic showed a BFN (or "big fat negative" as it's known in the fertility world). I am making light of things here, but after listening to the phone message from the clinic a few hours after the blood test, we were both pretty devastated.

We cried together in our kitchen and tried to process it. We both felt pretty numb. After dinner we just needed to get out of the house. We were profoundly exhausted, and I have to assume that Hope was even more exhausted than I was, having to go through the physical side too. We looked for a bar, café, or some space to escape to. It was raining hard as it tends to do in Ontario at the end of April. We eventually found a quaint, relaxing coffee lounge. The only patrons were two young people furiously typing away on their laptops with headphones.

Perfect, I thought.

The ambiance was mindfully relaxing and there were shelves full of books all around us, all with positive themes. We picked up different ones and started to read them separately whilst sitting next to each other. We shared pieces that spoke to us in that moment—our minds searching for meaning, for sense, for some promising sense direction.

The Book of Awesome by Neil Parsricha helped lift our spirits just by thinking about something else for a change in a humorous way. There was a book of affirmations and one of those *Chicken Soup for the Soul* books aimed at mothers with a hundred short stories. One story dealt with a couple in a similar situation to us who even named their children they could not have. In this story dreams did not die, they only took different forms and turned out to still deliver what they wanted, just not the way it might have been predicted, which restored the couple's faith in destiny and love and faith and hope. It did that for us too.

SOON THEREAFTER I STARTED THINKING ABOUT THE adoption process again and sent a message to the adoption agency to explain that it had been two years since we started the process and had not heard anything from them and would they contact us with a status update. We had also decided to take a month off. Furthermore, because it was Hope's birthday month, we decided to take a week-long vacation—hell, she *really* deserved it, and it would give her body a chance to recuperate a bit.

We still had a lot of options at this point, yet it was important to take a step back and think carefully about how much energy we had. We had always dismissed the idea of in vitro fertilization (IVF), but after six unsuccessful IUI attempts, the expectation was the doctor would suggest this as the best step as the statistics suggest that, after six tries, the odds of IUI success start to fall off. Or rather the odds of success for couples who have tried six times are not considered good.

And there was a new wrinkle as well.

The Ontario provincial government had just approved one-time free IVF starting in 2015, but *that* was eight months away. Hope was about to turn thirty-six and at that age, she felt that eight months was a long time to squander. We were taking a month off, so that left seven months of potential cycles. We had tried four times in a row, and two times before that. At this point I did not know what to do. My suspicions were that we would try another IUI before reviewing the IVF option. In the meantime we'd just given the adoption pot another stir.

Now it was time to take a breather.

Twelve

I WONDER IF YOU EVER FIND THAT THE MOMENT YOU take a break from a long stint at work with no vacation is the very moment that your body decides to become ill. Well, we didn't get so much physically ill, but our spirits were pretty crushed, and I am convinced that the slew of negative incidents that followed were related to where we were at.

It made me ask myself a lot of questions: How were we going to look after ourselves and maintain a sense of sanctuary in the aftermath of the last disappointment? Well, we could leave, but it would just follow us. We were going to stay right where we were. We had worked very hard trying to find a place to call home and had built the right set-up and spent a lot of time, energy, and money to create not just a house but a home.

So what options did we have to manage staying here in this home? One option would be to carry on as usual. Another would be to do that and also consider some landscaping options either inside or out, so we would have a "newness" to our home. Another option would be to put up some feng shui supports to encourage the anger and other demons that I had to flow through and out of the house. With this energy in my heart, it was not conducive to relaxing and feeling tranquil when trying to conceive.

One element that had been really stressful and not at all conducive to conception was the timing required to get to the cycle monitoring in the morning and then to get to work afterwards. The follow-up appointment with the doctor had included a consult asking for a longer consult! How pointless is that? The options presented to us were to do IVF or to step up the aggressiveness with the drugs on the next cycle. I was not completely happy that these were presented as our only choices, so we started to consider a different clinic. We looked at different clinics, in particular, ones near where Hope worked. The latter option seemed to make more sense—to go to the one near where Hope worked so she could relax and we could take our time whilst there.

All of these sporadic considerations were culminating in a sense of sadness, disappointment, and frustration, and as a result I felt down and less engaged with the rest of my life. I found out that my job was potentially not that secure as a result of a snap election on the horizon, the outcome of which my position depended upon. What was going to happen would directly influence our family and family-making options. There were a lot of potential changes around the corner, and I felt a deep need to feel grounded again and reflect on what was really important and strategize how to manage it all. We had booked a week off together and decided it would be a good time to meditate with nature—an opportunity to get away and reflect on what we wanted and how we were going to manage the turning fortunes of time. This was a good time to breathe and review our lives and what we wanted for them.

WE SET OFF ON OUR PLANNED WEEK OFF, SPENDING the first day and night at a family member's farm. Having that immediate relief from changing the surroundings revealed the negative energy that had been surrounding me. This highlighted for me the choices around how we choose to perceive things versus acknowledging and accepting how things affect us. I had to accept that I was indeed incredibly pissed off by the bullshit this process had caused us.

A part of me wondered about patience being a virtue and the idea that this difficult time in my life would pass. Another part of me, however, felt incredibly sad that the whole range of angry emotions I was experiencing daily just seemed so pointless and unnecessary.

This first vacation day was a good one, and helped me see the difference in how I was responding to being surrounded by nature, family, and loving energy. It was also Hope's thirty-sixth birthday, which was both triggering and bittersweet. I say triggering because thirty-six is considered the age at which pregnancy starts to become just that little bit more difficult. We had booked a conversation with the fertility doctor we were seeing the following weekend, and had just been referred to another fertility clinic nearer to where Hope worked. The day we returned to the fertility clinic after our vacation would be day three of Hope's cycle, and another potential try at IUI.

The following day, off we went, early in the morning, to Tobermory, Ontario. It was a beautiful drive, and a beautiful day for a trip. We arrived and had lunch and strolled around the lazy marine town and dropped into the visitor centre. Despite a good start to the day, I could feel a nagging frustration and anger starting to swell inside of me. Mindful of this, I tried to fight it and remain present and hopeful. We both needed the rest, relaxation, and recuperation—we needed a renewed sense of positivity and hope for the future.

We had a half-hour evening walk and visited a lookout tower that was both calming and quiet. It felt like the wind was blowing away my thoughts though I could still feel this nagging anger inside of me. We went walking and rode a glass-bottom boat to see shipwrecks, a welcomed hour of escape. This was followed by a grossly overpriced severely nutrient-lacking lunch, which was a double whammy of frustration for me: I cannot stand wasting money, and I feel physically shitty when putting shit food into my body.

Still, we were on vacation. I was trying desperately hard to recognize how incredibly grateful I was that we were eating at all, as many people could not, and that we could afford it as many people cannot. The time away was causing me to get really caught up with my own thoughts and feelings. At least at home there were distractions, routines, house maintenance, chores, errands, the gym, work, people, friends, family to focus on. Now all that was gone. On vacation, life is lived moment-by-moment, experience and decisions made based on how we felt. It was intense.

One of the days we were away it rained hard and got really cold, and for a time it seemed like we were not going to end up doing too much. But eventually it stopped, and we went off around Tobermory. We bought a bottle of wine and took it back to the room, but the bag snapped and the bottle shattered, the red wine pool everywhere like blood. It gave a bleeding heart visual to my inside world. I cleaned up and threw it all out and felt an emptiness afterwards.

Now with no wine to relax, off we went for a hike. It turned out to be not as long as I had hoped—maybe an hour and a half maximum—and with my state of mind as dark as it was I felt ripped off and not very accomplished at all. What it was doing for me, however, was helping me notice that I had this innate need to keep moving, to keep feeling like I was moving *towards* something. I could not sit in my depression. And that revealed to me why I was applying for another job, feeling the need to run, feeling the need to move homes. I would meet challenges and issues with movement and action, and if I didn't, I would feel this deep sense of angst, of frustration and anger. And the flames of that anger were being fanned by my sense of not being in control. This was anger smouldering in my perception of things not happening the way I believed they should be happening—*should* being a particularly inflammatory concept.

Yes sir, I was definitely angry.

Angry at myself, angry at work, angry at being infertile, angry at God, angry at life, angry at the world—the news made me angry. I was angry at the thought of Nigerian schoolgirls being raped in the jungle, at the stories of the millions of Syrians killed and villages savaged. I was angry that five years after a massive earthquake, most Haitians were still suffering in camps. Angry at the wars in the Ukraine, the Middle East, and God knows where else. I was angry what seemed like a global epidemic of human rights violations. My faith was shot. My heart was broken, and I wanted a get out plan. But I could not leave.

This is what started me to move towards the idea of trying IVF. The tricky thing was that, even if it were to be covered—and I wasn't naïve enough to think *that* was a done deal—it would not come into effect until the following year. And in the meantime that meant at least seven other tries to conceive passing us by.

That day, in Tobermory, was when my thinking started to shift towards the possibility of us trying IVF and the realization that, if we did, it was likely going to involve paying for it—which meant around $20,000. The only decision it seemed to me was the date and the clinic. Would we try the new clinic? And with a two-month wait liest, that would mean July at the earliest and more likely August, for they would likely want to do a month of cycle monitoring first. And August would bring us to within four months of it being covered. Could we wait? *Should* we wait? I didn't have any of answers. What I had was a strong desire to scream. I was so fucking angry.

THE NEXT DAY WE WERE GOING TO GODERICH, AND although it's a place famed for being the most beautiful place in the province—my kind of place—I was starting to suspect that the next few days were not going to be good days. I was trying to recognize that these feelings needed coming out and that having this time off was giving them space to come out. Looking back, I think it was good to create that space for that anger to emerge. It felt fucking awful and incredibly uncomfortable, and I hated every fucking second of it.

On the way home I started to recognize that there was a brewing amount of unfair resentment churning away inside me. I think it was a blessing that there had always been this ongoing difference between Hope and I around how we cope with disappointment and feeling out of control. I was learning more about my overin-flated sense of righteousness. You may find this when you have been striving as a team for a long time to achieve something that's not happening and you feel like you *deserve* it. The difficult feelings that you have no time to sit with all start to surface the moment you have a break. I had been exercising and throwing myself into work to try and distract myself from these difficult feelings. Now, with a break from both, they were all I had left to sit with.

Thirteen

HOPE'S PERSONALITY IS DIFFERENT FROM MINE, and thank God for that. Neither personality is right or wrong, they just are what they are. All of this is fine, of course, and we both accept the other's tendencies. I recognized that my anger—the main feeling I had been left sitting with post vacation—was not something I had a lot of good techniques to manage. I saw my anger as a mask for a deeper anxiety and feelings of hopelessness at not being able to control our childlessness.

We booked an appointment with a naturopath to try and look at ways to improve the health and well-being of our situation beyond Western medicine. We were prescribed diaries and supplements and different references for support. We reminisced about how humbling it had been to not get pregnant and mused that if the our present selves could tell our past selves this, then perhaps we would not have been so unarmored and vulnerable at our early disappointments! The naturopath recommended focusing on our well-being and taking a break of two to three months from fertility appointments to get into a better state. I was feeling a building emptiness inside of me without children. It seemed folks who had kids were seeing the important stuff of life—a profound experience of being connected to life, and yes, the challenges only having children could bring. I was feeling bored with the monotony of my own overly-free life.

I had to get out of the house to stop myself from articulating these damaging statements in front of Hope. I had to walk out and get some air and space. I ended up walking around the neighbourhood each morning and swearing to myself. Of course, this was all the built-up anger talking, and it was feeding off of the infertility, which was a food I could not starve it from. I love Hope, and there are very few things more distressing in this world than watching someone you love in a crap load of pain when there is nothing you can do about it and you are, in your own way, unintentionally contributing to it because you cannot produce the one thing you might biologically expect a person like me to be able to.

AFTER A COUPLE OF MONTHS, WE DECIDED TO GO IN for one final consult with our doctor at the clinic, and that's when we began to speak about IVF. Towards the end of that consult, the doctor mentioned that it might be possible to put us in for a clinical trial named AUGMENT℠ treatment, a Canadian-approved process, which would mean we get our IVF paid for. I was not expecting this and it totally threw me off-guard.

Oh my God, that's amazing!

But almost immediately the doctor had to hedge the suggestion because she realized there was an age restriction—and we were just on the cusp of it. If we turned out to not qualify for the trial then that would be a real mind fuck for me. Perhaps it was just a way for the doctor to soften the blow and give us a bit of hope and support. Many doctors we have experienced have an inability to be empathetic and supportive emotionally. I imagine that is at least partly because of the realities of a system where time equals money and the need trying to balance that out with quality care. It also seems like certain specialties attract a certain type of personality. Let me just leave that statement at that.

Going through something like fertility issues is about endurance. To push through something when you don't believe it's ever going to change is incredibly difficult. Giving up is easy by comparison, and you are faced with that option at almost every turn. You may decide to give up for a moment or for the day or a few months—or forever. Another option is that you may decide to keep going despite not seeing an answer or believing it is going to make a difference to your circumstances. Either way, you are going to make a choice and it will be your choice. No matter how it may appear to others, it is your choice. You are deciding for yourself how to handle the situation you are in. Giving up might be running away; at the same time, giving up might be self-care. That part is a fine line that only you can discern by gauging how you are feeling and trying to stay as in touch and authentic with yourself as possible. Like any kind of fight, only you know where your personal tipping points are. You need to push yourself to those points and be willing to reassess every time you get there.

WE SPENT THE REST OF DAY AWAY FROM EACH OTHER in order to know our own minds. This whole journey was becoming so much bigger than failed attempts at procreation—it was about bearing witness to something that was laying us both bare. We had been with each other for extended periods of time in deeply intimate circumstances as needed in this kind of journey, and isolated from other relationships which are vital in life-including independent relationships with ourselves. Knowing that one is alone at times and has a degree of spaciousness from others is not enough. You have to tend and nurture that space as part of daily practice. I am pretty confident it is a universal human experience.

Luckily, because we are all so diverse and try different ways to strive to improve the quality of human existence both externally and within, it can be helpful to see what has worked for someone else. It became helpful to support each other with the idea that there was no harm in trying an array of actions to see which one fit better.

It's up to each person to take ownership of their self-care, otherwise one will keep losing things and losing *at* things. I perceived that we were losing time, money, energy, opportunities and moments of happiness and peace in life. I had to take care of myself and recognize that. Taking myself out of the house seemed to be the only thing that made sense. It afforded me the time and space to focus and take stock of the energies available to me.

I knew I would have to proactively connect with others in my community. I would have to consider how I was going to take care of myself and muster new resources and strategies if I were going to affect anything transformative.

I spent the next three weeks sleeping in a separate room. This was not about discord but rather an exercise in creating the space for me to process my own thoughts and feelings. I filled almost every evening with a social event or at least being out of the house after dinner and doing some writing or reading at a local coffee shop.

June was warm in the evenings, good running weather. When I ran, I did so with the intention of self-betterment not only for my own sake and the sake of my marriage, but for the sake of my future children. This would be the environment and habits they would be brought into. A space where it would be secure enough to have time away, yet enjoyable enough when together, to have deeper connection that did not suffocate the other or cause co-dependent dynamics or social ostracism.

During this time, I perceived personal insecurities that stemmed from my history, mainly financial insecurity—more so in my mind than in reality—coupled with my insecure attachment to the idea of independence and the need not to rely on anyone else in my life. Both of these insecurities were causing me to disconnect from myself, and I had lost myself in dedication to work and other pursuits. That, I recognized, is not what life—at least not a happy sustainable life—was about, at least not for me.

Of course, all this soul searching doesn't mean that our fertility struggles had been put on hold. Quite the opposite. But wait, I've wandered somewhat into the background here.

Let's rewind a bit, shall we?

Fourteen

OKAY, SO WE'D COME BACK FROM TOBERMORY, AND at the suggestion of a naturopath, had taken a little time off to gather our wits and recuperate from the rigours and disappointments we'd already faced.

It was late May 2014.

We had a scheduled consultation at the clinic because now, after six unsuccessful IUI attempts, there were a lot of factors to consider. We went in and, for the most part, were not really told anything we had not already researched ourselves. Then, as I mentioned earlier, just as we were gearing up to leave, we were informed that we may qualify for a clinical trial for a new procedure called AUGMENT^{SM} treatment, which was being approved by Health Canada, and intended to augment the ova's ability to sustain itself through mitochondria precursor cells—the energy making systems of a cell—in utero when fertilized via IVF. The next sentence was the real complete shocker

"...and of course as part of a clinical trial, you would get your procedure covered."

When I heard this it was like time slowed down, and I felt a tingle of excitement in my body again. I'm sure it showed on Hope's face as well as mine.

"Yes, but hold on. You may not qualify as there is an age cut-off for this trial, and you folks would be right on the cusp."

Hmm, can we say mind fuck?

Hope was on board immediately and wanted the doctor to enquire about this on our behalf. And so we left the clinic feeling very... strange! I think we really didn't know how to feel. We both referred to this sensation as "like being on a rollercoaster" at some point of the car journey home.

Strangely, just thirty minutes earlier, we were about to divorce that clinic altogether and try a new one. Now we were considering doing an IVF cycle with the same clinic!

ABOUT FIVE DAYS LATER, WE GOT THE CALL TO SAY we qualified for the trial. This felt like a true miracle in so many ways. It made us both believe even more so in the idea of the Law of Attraction: where you put out to the universe what you desire and it brings it to you in the form that you need to see it. Having this procedure covered meant it would cost between five and six thousand dollars as opposed to sixteen to eighteen thousand dollars, a *substantial* difference. The costs we would being paying would cover the drugs involved in the procedure and—we had coverage for most of the cost of these drugs. We knew that we were truly blessed, for many folks do not have this privilege. Now we were suddenly on a path to trying something brand new. We had never anticipated or even allowed ourselves to contemplate such an opportunity.

The procedure that made this a clinical trial instead of a regular IVF cycle was the fact that it involved day surgery on the ovaries in advance of the cycle itself. The procedure would perform a biopsy on the ovary and extract mitochondria precursor cells, which would then be stored and injected into the ova that would be used in the IVF cycle. The hypothesis as, far as we were told, was that the extra mitochondrial energy would mean increased success rates. The potential for this would be the development of a very powerful process for infertile couples—not to mention huge business for pharmaceuticals. So it would start with day surgery. Now we just had to wait for the call.

Hope was a real trooper. She had already been through so much physically. As the partner I was hyper-aware of this and felt I had to be strong and stoic the whole time. A friend of mine shared with me that I needed to learn how to be vulnerable and become more okay about being less in control. So I tried to spend more time being fancy-free. I was beginning to recognize it was important to stay grounded and diligent in taking better care of my own well-being. I needed to remember that I was a decent person, and I was trying to be wise in my choices, behaviours, decisions and responses to others. I used meditation a lot to help remain conscious in my relationship, which was critically important.

Hope said that it was like we were dating all over again. We were starting to become unstuck because we were liberating ourselves, so when we were together it was more magical. It had stagnated because we had had to spend so much time together in our private mission to become parents. Hope had finally shared with her parents what we had been trying to accomplish for last year and a half. We had both ignorantly thought, at the beginning, that we would have been successful by now. I had envisioned that we would be sharing the news of a pregnancy with them through a grandparent greeting card. Instead we were sharing our failed attempts in order to draw upon support and understanding of loving relatives to renew our hope and sense of not being so alone in the journey.

WE GOT THE CALL ABOUT THE AUGMENTˢᴹ **TREAT-**ment at the beginning of June and were told that the process was to start at the end of August. That was perfect because it meant that we had about two and a half months to really enjoy the summer and get into healthier individual habits. It would also afford us some breathing space before embarking again on the baby-making journey.

We had been so focused on this aspect of life that there had not been much time or consideration for other relationships. I was spending more time with some amazing friends and family members, something I had not done in a long while. I was starting to achieve a better balance between work, social life and home life. I was starting to enjoy life more. At first I put it down to the weather being warmer, allowing me to get outside. But I think you might find that it's absolutely crucial to keep those friends and family close to you even if you don't take a few months off—even if it's just in between the clinic appointments and inseminations and waiting periods. It's easy when you and your partner are going through something like this to simply dig a two-person foxhole, and that's not healthy.

When I reflect on why I didn't do this earlier, I certainly think the money aspect had something to do with it. I almost did not want to give myself permission to go out and have a good time because we were going to be down an indefinite amount of money and, let's be honest here, a social life requires optional expenses. The problem is that cutting some corners in order to save money gives rise to hidden costs of a different kind.

Spending money that you can "afford"—albeit in large scary arbitrary chunks—can admittedly lead to debt. But reasonable monetary debt is recoverable with planning and time. Having a mental breakdown, however, is potentially not so recoverable no matter how much time and planning happens. It was time to budget more holistically.

I had always had a baseline insecurity when it came to money. One of the things I had learned since we'd started pursuing pregnancy was that, when it came to money, my fear of the issue was bigger than the issue itself. Money could be saved and spent if need be. We were already more than ten thousand dollars in the hole with nothing (other than the experience itself) to show for it. And yet the sky had not fallen. That in and of itself was a valuable lesson.

Another lesson learned was that time marched forward. It never pauses or slows just because things aren't going your way. When you start thinking about children, it inevitably, and naturally, leads to thinking of your own mortality. Hope and I could save money; we knew that now. We could recover expenses. But no one can recover months unlived. Lost time is lost forever. If we were going to have children it would be more important to leave them wisdom gleaned from experience and healthy examples of balanced lives than it would be to leave them money.

You can become addicted to saving, but life is for living—and we had a summer of it ahead of us.

Fifteen

OUR SUMMER OFF WAS CUT SHORT, HOWEVER, IN July when we were called to drop everything and come into the clinic a month earlier because there had been a cancellation. We were caught off guard and had lots of questions, for which we got very few satisfying answers. One thing should be made clear though; in situations like this, you always have the option to stick with your original dates. You do not have to step up to fill a cancellation. Do not be afraid that if you do not take that cancellation you'll be dropped. You won't be.

We got another call shortly thereafter suggesting that we may after all not be covered. If we were not covered, then that would give us closure. It would provide us with closure to these ridiculous back and forth antics—and the opportunity to start over knowing what we would look for in a new clinic. Either way it would be a positive step forward. Though framing it like this was perhaps a mind game we used to feel more in control. Hey, my view is to help yourself by doing whatever you need to do—so long as it doesn't hurt you or someone else— in order to keep your sense of self in this crazy-making journey.

Not surprisingly, Hope was incredibly graceful and grounded through all of this. I don't know how she did it. Our unexpected trip to the clinic was frustrating and maddening. Hours spent needlessly waiting in rooms. Miscommunications. Vague half answers that raised more questions than they answered. But Hope kept her cool. At the clinic, she asked questions, would not be pushed into sign consent forms without reading them, and challenged the system when necessary.

I spent much of my time biting my tongue and making detailed notes for a client feedback survey that, when all was said and done, never materialized. (In the end I sent it as an unsolicited document.) The gist of my argument was that if patient stress suppresses the chances of conception then a lot of what was going on at this damned clinic was undermining what they were trying to achieve.

Part of the eight-page consent form they were trying to get us to sign was a detailed description of the procedures, policies, and the whole approach of what this research initiative was all about. It's important that all of this be clear to you and that if you don't understand something—if it seems too technical or deliberately vague—you ask questions.

The process had been put to us, in May, as a clinical trial, but it turned out to be more of a training process for the clinic's staff in order to hone the skillsets required to do this intra-cytoplasmic precursor cell injection procedure independently. This wasn't a deal-breaker but it simply hadn't been our initial understanding of the situation.

Luckily, at the bottom of the second to last page was name of the lead physician and a phone number with an invitation to call with any questions we might have about the procedure. *Bingo!* Here was the opportunity to regain some autonomy and independence within this situation through a process of enquiry.

It was Hope who called, and she asked exactly what we wanted to know: What is it about? Are we included? Are we covered? Is it safe? What are the rates of success?

The doctor was pleasantly approachable and, as it turns out, was actually part of another fertility clinic that had been recommended to us. So in one way, we were technically moving towards being treated by another clinic through this process, which pleased me, because it felt like trying something different and made me feel less insane. The doctor was able to say that, yes, our doctor had asked for an additional patient to be covered and that this must be us. This really helped both of us to feel empowered, even though we still needed to wait for confirmation from our own clinic later that week.

As it turns out, the clinic called a mere couple of hours later, twice leaving us a message to confirm both our inclusion and our coverage. This felt like we were regaining a sense of empowerment and an ability to navigate the system. The clinic had to step up and communicate better with the patients. It really didn't seem to be that difficult. We were extremely grateful that the doctor from the new clinic was actually talking to us like human beings and welcoming these patient interactions as part of the process of providing health care. What a concept!

WE WERE BOTH VERY PRIVILEGED TO BE ABLE TO easily book time off from work to mentally prepare for what lay ahead. I read up a lot on this new procedure and Hope and I even watched an amazing YouTube video we found. It's amazing what is out there these days if you sit down at a keyboard and look.

We got a call from the clinic prepping us for the laparoscopic surgery. They told us that, although they had originally given us a surgery date of August 25, we needed to be ready to go on July 25 and even cautioned us that, if we didn't comply, it might not happen at all.

What the FUCK are they talking about?

I'd just about had it with this clinic. The one promising conversation had been with the lead physician (from another clinic), but that's not who we were talking to now. I have to say I was ready to do some serious "advocacy" at this point, and Hope was getting stressed over whether to stand our ground or simply to adjust our sails accordingly to the system's fickle unfocussed winds.

Part of the problem is that it is all but impossible to figure out when folks are just being officious and provider-centric and when it is *genuinely* a limited access thing. Either way we knew we could miss our chance if we balked. In the end, we were told that if we didn't submit to the sudden date change, it wasn't happening. There are situations where you need to keep your head rather than blow up. It's important at moments like this to take your time, breathe, and talk with each other. You *generally* have more choices than you think.

As distressing and infuriating as it was, we took the newer date. It was confirmed in short order, and Hope was then qualified and booked. We never did get a solid explanation of any sort as to what the hell was going on. We decided to let it go, as this was the sort of bullshit that could drive people crazy. And we knew that stress was something we had to manage. That being said, all this was added to my growing "survey notes."

Sixteen

JULY 25, 2014 WAS A FRIDAY. WE HAD BOTH TAKEN the day off of work and had gone into the city early enough to avoid the rush hour traffic. Originally we'd been told that Hope's laparoscopic surgery was scheduled for 7:30 a.m., which would have worked out fine for us. Unfortunately, we'd been called the night before at 10 p.m. (we were already in bed due to early morning we were facing) and informed that we'd been bumped back three hours. Fine. There was no point arguing and no point leaving later only to get mired in traffic, so it meant more waiting once we arrived.

We had coffee and waited. Fast forward to Hope and I sitting patiently in a waiting room, Hope in a hospital gown. She then got called in and was asked first to take her glasses off and give them to me. Then, half-blind, she was asked to follow the porter, who then decided to kill two birds with one stone and take *another* patient, at the same time, to the intensive care unit on a bed, along with all this patient's family. So there was Hope in nothing but a hospital gown padding barefoot after this guy as part of an entourage of strangers. You can't make this stuff up.

This too went into my notes.

I didn't see Hope again for six hours. Eventually I was approached by the doctor who did the surgery and was told that it had been a relatively good procedure and that Hope looked all good inside and just had a little bit of bleeding on her left side. She also told me how long it would be until I'd see her again, so I had a chance to go get something to eat and some fresh air. I was grateful for that. I treated myself to a twenty-dollar sandwich—I kid you not—from the hospital cafeteria.

When I got called in to see Hope, I was handed a prescription and told to go get it filled out at the hospital pharmacy, for it would take Hope a while to recuperate enough to be discharged. It was expected to take one hour, but it was an additional six hours before she was ready to leave. I think the drugs really knocked her out, and the staff wouldn't let her leave until they were sure she was all good. Thirty-two dollars later, we were out of the parking lot. We were grateful for the successful procedure and grateful for the chance to have been able to have tried it. We were grateful that, by the grace of God, it was covered under this research trial. If only hospital sandwiches and parking were covered.

A follow-up meeting was to be scheduled four to six weeks later, but after what was a needless rigmarole—though sadly typical with this particular clinic—trying to nail down a date, we were eventually told not to bother.

"...just come in for your next cycle, and we'll start the process."

At that point, Hope's next cycle meant that the process would start mid-September and would involve hormone treatment to produce more eggs.

LATE AUGUST. IT WAS AROUND TWO WEEKS BEFORE the try and our second wedding anniversary. It had been a rollercoaster journey in the short time we had been married. We had known each other for eleven years and had been together for seven. The fertility journey had been a great chance for us to really understand and know each other and love each other deeply in so many different ways, and support each other as we had in previous difficult times too. From my experience, going through a stressful time is so often the litmus test of a sincere and lasting connection with someone. It had been a lovely summer, and we had enjoyed it immensely. We had reflected that not only was late August around this time of year we had married, it was also this time of year we had gotten together, and the time of year we had first met in Japan all those years ago. Now it was the time we were going to make children. This was our time of year. This was *our* time. Our time.

I had read a lot and listened to the experience of other women who'd gone through this process. It sounded harsh, as you might expect. Putting a human body through a forced hyper-stimulation process is stressful. So I had to be prepared if I was going to be a proper support. I was focused and repeating a mantra to myself daily: *Be patient, be kind, be understanding.* I was focused on creating a space for Hope to vent and be irritable, outlandish, extreme—literally all the things that we were doing to her body. I understood that there would be passing behaviours in response to the battle going on inside her body. Hope apologized to me in advance, and I told her she had a free license to order as much poutine as she wanted! Yes, I am a committed partner, and we were in this together. Since I could not experience these things directly for Hope, I would try my best to be there for her and help her let her stress out physically through exercise, verbally through conversation, behaviourally through whatever she needed to do.

Short of harmful activities, as far as I was concerned, she had carte blanche. She'd earned it.

My mum was going to come visit that month. The last time we'd tried was the last time she'd been over to visit. I so desperately wanted her to become a grandmother, especially in this time of her life. She was in such good place and also about to retire. She knew, this time around, what was happening and it would likely be a good distraction for us to have her there. I had a lot of great people around me, people I connected or reconnected with over the previous six months. They were so incredibly supportive and had helped me believe in myself more.

WHEN WE RETURNED TO THE CLINIC IN MID-SEPTEM- ber, Hope was told that she'd need to self-inject twice a day with various hormones (Menopur, Bravelle, and other concoctions). As the support partner, I figured the least I could do was perform the scary injections. It is bad enough having to be injected, but self-injection is worse—there is a lot of gearing up that has to be done especially if you are doing multiple injections a day.

I fell even deeper in love with Hope when I saw again how brave and courageous she really was. I learned to inject her daily with these hormones. I would put the vials under my armpit at 6:30 a.m. to warm up the oil-submerged drug to body temperature and then prepare the needles—there was one for drawing up and another for injecting so as to keep the tip sharp at the moment of skin puncture. A quick alcohol wipe of her stomach, and a conversation topic to re-direct her attention away from the injection, and we got ourselves into a bit of a routine.

Hope responded quickly to the drugs—bloating, cramping, thirst and tiredness. Of course, it's an emotionally tumultuous situation, so it's kind of hard to tell sometimes what the heck is causing what symptom. As the vessel, Hope had to make sure she transported herself to the clinic regularly for an ongoing series of progress assessments, ultrasounds and blood tests to check her hormone levels and egg development.

By day six we had three eggs.

We had heard several stories of people who had managed to get *dozens* and so we were not too sure what to make of this. By day nine, we had six eggs and were told this was good for her age. By day thirteen it was time to aspirate them. Yes, aspirate, like she's some kind of test tube or well-aged wine. I really did not like the way the system dehumanized her. Some doctors were better at recognizing and compensating for the lingo than others. Unfortunately, the most frequent experience was that of being choo-chooed along on the fertility train. It felt very patronizing.

Before being booked for the aspiration process, there was, *of course*, another set of consent forms. This set was nine pages long and—I kid you not—when we had questions we were told by the doctor to "make it quick."

Nice, right?

A lot of the questions on this form were ones that we had not anticipated. They covered topics such as what we'd agree to do with extra eggs, extra sperm, and any extra embryos; questions like whether we'd allow the clinic to take some for research or donate them to other people. These are big questions, worthy of some thought and discussion.

"Make it quick."

Don't be bullied. Take your time.

With forms signed, and with six eggs ready to go, we were booked for 7 a.m. the next morning. We decided to make an adventure of it and were up around 4:45 a.m. and travelling into Toronto to beat the traffic. This process was so time sensitive that we literally had to drop everything to prioritize it. Of course, you don't find out until a day or so beforehand what day it will be. Luckily by now Hope had told her boss what was going on in our lives—she had to for her own sake. All the sick days and sense of anxiety it was causing trying to cover it up was getting to be very stressful in itself.

We arrived at the clinic, and almost immediately Hope got hooked up to all sorts of wires and was administered multiple drugs. One of the medications was to calm her, another one to manage her blood pressure, and yet another to sedate her. Fortunately, we had a good doctor who was very professional and supportive, and he gave us the rundown of what to expect. Healthcare providers take note, *this* is extremely helpful to the overall experience! We were to expect a procedure that was to take five minutes or less.

With Hope on a bed, and me in scrubs, we went into the procedure room and Hope assumed the position. The ultrasound picks up solid mass as white and fluid as black—that's how it is translated onto the screen. So for each follicle sac that had a potential egg inside, it showed up as a black space on the screen. With that in place, the doctor went through a catheter into the uterus, penetrating the uterine and ovarian wall to pierce each follicle and aspirate all the fluid along with the egg inside.

The team managed to get five of the six follicles that were there, and for every egg that was aspirated, there was a huge counter on the wall of the room beeping the number each time. It was a neon sign like the ones you might see at a delicatessen as you are waiting your turn for your ticket to be called. Hope seemed to be in pain but was managing it well, knowing it was going to be very temporary.

Once we were done, we left the operating room to return to the recovery room, and she slept for about forty-five minutes. Whilst sitting there, watching her, I could see how lucky I was to have such a beautiful, brave, wonderful person sharing this journey with me, and I felt so honoured.

We could hear the doctor having a conversation with another patient in the next room and how they had retrieved twenty-seven eggs! Immediately Hope and I felt deflated—but we kept telling ourselves that it was quality not quantity. I do know that there is some truth to that, I was just not sure how much. Besides, there was nothing more we could do about the number of eggs. Instead our attention turned immediately, upon discharge, to commencing the intramuscular injections of progesterone.

These were done to promote the uterine lining forming which would also prevent potential miscarriage. The regimen now was to take antibiotics and wait for a phone call from the clinic every couple of days regarding how the eggs were doing, whilst at the same time, administering these shots to Hope. The most anxiety provoking call was the first one. We had gone back to work the day of the procedure and had to wait all day to be able to listen to the voice message the clinic left.

All five eggs had matured, and all five had fertilized.

We both dropped to the floor and wept with relief, knowing that we could let go for now.

That night we told ourselves over and over that it was quality not quantity that counted, and that had certainly proved to be true by the results thus far. The wait, however, over next few days made us both incredibly anxious. Administering the progesterone shots was intense enough, but we also were on edge waiting to receive a call (time of day undetermined and seemingly random) from the clinic. That call would give us an update on the status of how the now fertilized eggs were doing and thus our chances at the point of transfer back inside Hope—if any of them would make it to that point.

It felt profound to know that, at this point in time, we had gotten further than we ever had before. And we held, in our hearts, the knowledge that five embryos were alive. Five of my Hope's eggs had been fertilized and were living on this Earth; it was an incredible thought. In order to distract ourselves, and with my mum in town too, we went out to museums and galas galore to pass the time. We even dropped into a 3.9-million-dollar open house my sister-in-law's company was staging just to live in fantasy land for a few hours.

Whilst sitting down in a field (well, in a gazebo in a field) mid-afternoon, we got the next call. We were told that all five fertilized eggs were dividing and that the clinic had assigned a figure on a number system for both the number of cells each embryo had divided into and their graded quality. It turns out that each clinic does this scoring differently, but this clinic graded them one to five, with one being the best. We had five embryos. Three had divided into two cells and showing a quality of grade two; one embryo at four cells with a quality of grade three; and one embryo at five cells showing a quality of grade two. We were experiencing all new feelings with this—mostly uncertainty, for with no comparators, we were not really too sure what to make of those numbers. All we knew really was that it was working so far.

The following day we got a call at a different time with the same update regimen. This time we were told they were growing a little slower but that all were growing.

In between each call, we spent hours on Google searching for hopeful comments and also educating ourselves. Why? Because our clinic had not provided us with any consultation as to what these numbers were like in comparison to the general IVF population. Without context the numbers being reported to us meant very little.

When you're the recipient of such an invasive and personal process as this, please remember that you have the right to ask as many bloody questions as you bloody well please. Looking back, I wish we had demanded more answers. Seriously, if the providers push back to stop you in any way when you ask questions, just mention the OMA [Ontario Medical Association] or RNAO [Registered Nurses' Association of Ontario] and their respective complaints commissions. Tell them that you know your rights to be fully informed. Tell them that it is their responsibility to keep you informed, so you're doing them a favour by covering their ass.

By day three we were told that, although they were not growing as the doctor would like, we would be asked to come back to the clinic downtown for the transfer on day five, and at that point, we would be told how many would be recommended for transfer. Now at this point I was again incredibly proud of Hope who simply called the lab directly, got through to the embryologist, and was informed that there would likely be three viable fertilized eggs to be transferred.

That was helpful information because it meant we had some time—albeit 24 hours—to make a decision as to how many embryos to transfer and how many to freeze. We decided, up front, that we would like to transfer two—if it worked and we got twins that would be a bonus! We thought it would be an option to then freeze the third.

DAY FIVE, THE DAY OF TRANSFER WAS UPON US.

Again, we are called in to get downtown as early as possible to be ready to transfer by 7 a.m., which meant a 4:45 wake up. Remember, there had also been daily progesterone shots, and we were doing this before leaving the house on the day of the transfer also. Hope had been so brave with so many invasive procedures and relinquishing control of this whole process.

We arrived, and the doctor was singing out pop songs and talking at great length about her own children. Though I was happy for her to be so positive about her own parenthood, we did not want to hear it, we wanted and needed support and guidance about our own present moment struggles.

I tried to distract and redirect Hope to visualize our trip to Cuba—the sand, sea and sun—and recall how relaxed she might have felt as we prepared for the final procedure. When the doctor checked in with us, we asked what the status was of the embryos. The doctor hadn't read up on the notes prior to talking with us, as we knew more than she did, which was quite an eye opener given such a critical moment. We got called in and prepared for the transfer. Then, just as Hope was in stirrups, ready for the transfer, that was the moment the doctor decided to (a) reinforce how wonderful her own children were, (b) tell us the embryos looked crap and were unlikely to work, and (c) recommended putting in all three and forget about freezing anything.

Thus, in one fell three-second swoop, the complexion of everything had changed. We were then handed a form for Hope to sign *immediately* as the doctor stood over her with the syringe. At this point her legs were up in stirrups, she was half naked, with multiple people looking over her. She'd just been given shitty information and afforded no time to process it.

"Here, sign this."

Yes, this *actually* happened.

I was so angry at the lack of empathy and awareness of the medical model being conducted here, but I did not have time to look at that anger. So I told Hope to look at me, and *only* me, and to then close her eyes and think about good times we had had on Varadero beach, and how beautiful the blue ocean was and how it gave a sense of peace and serenity.

In the background, the embryologist asked the doctor permission to "hatch" the embryos, which means he was weakening the outer shell to help them become ready for implantation once they reach the blastocyst stage, if they made it that far. The blastocyst stage is what we wanted them to ideally be by now, but they couldn't stay outside the body any longer. The blastocyst stage is when the cells are starting to differentiate, and under the microscope you can actually see an outer layer and inner layer of cells distinctly that are to become the placenta and the baby respectively. The hope was that they were just a little slow and, by this time tomorrow, after time growing inside of Hope, they would reach that stage. Once the transfer was done, a few minutes later, we were out of there.

There is a lot of information encouraging potential birth part-ners in this moment of their journey to try and relax as much as possible. There has been some anecdotal research that acupunc-ture just before and just after these procedures can help with this. Hope had had an acupuncture session just before going into the procedure that morning. Afterwards we drove home and went to her home naturopath for another acupuncture session. After that shitty experience that we had no control over, she deserved a little bit of support to help her relax.

THE NEXT TWO WEEKS WERE SPENT CONVINCING ourselves it had worked and giving ourselves a reason to stay positive and relaxed while keeping up with the progesterone injections. My mother returned home, and we went over to Hope's younger sister's place to celebrate her own pregnancy announce-ment. Of course we were both incredibly happy for her and her partner. Now two of the three sisters had become pregnant ! We were so happy that we were going to have another niece or nephew. We were never jealous. We were just more reflective of how profound and amazing it is when it does happen *anywhere* to *anyone* that wants it.

I can't lie—I was also feeling somewhat depressed that I couldn't give to Hope what we so wanted, no matter how hard we might try. We were constantly faced with the fact that it might never end up happening. I was bouncing in between different states—I would feel morose one day, and then the next day I would feel calm and content and accepting of whatever may come.

To cut a long story short—as you can see we are not at the end of this book *yet*—once again, no BFP [Big Fat Positive] for us. We had resisted testing early until the day of the blood test. That day it was a holiday. She tested negative on the pee stick, and six hours later, through the blood test results, we confirmed.

Not pregnant.

Hearing the result this time, I was calmer. I guess I was just use to it by now, and so was Hope. Later on the tears came.

Seventeen

PERHAPS ONE OF THE MOST SURREAL AND UNSET-
tling aspects of going through a particularly intense experience is
that time doesn't stop. Ever. It moves forward, and if you stop, it
marches on without you. The world moves on. It's a good lesson to
learn. Get back up. Keep moving.

Now we knew for certain that we were *never* going to go back
to this particular clinic again. I am not going to name it here, but
what I will say is, trust your own instincts when you are inter-
facing with any health care provider-if you do not feel heard,
respected or treated with integrity, do not waste any more of
your time or money there. There are many clinics out there, with
different cultures-find the one that works for you in your heart
first because that intuit sense is going to be your primary driver
along this journey. We knew we were going to choose to move on
from this mismatch. Hope had proactively kept an appointment
with another clinic that had a good reputation for patient-centred
care and wrote to the old clinic to transfer and make a copy of all
the medical records of all previous attempts. This way we could
start to gain control of the situation again. We were so much more
knowledgeable. We were going to this new appointment at this
new clinic, knowing more thoroughly what was going on. We had

also been through an IVF cycle to diagnose and understand additional problems more thoroughly. We knew now that IUIs were a waste of time and money for us. That is a crappy uncertainty you cannot know until you've done it for yourself and seen both how your partner's body responds to it and/or how many times you're willing and able to try.

We called the adoption services again and they said that we should get a call in the next few months for the training they deliver. They also pointed out that, in the initial paperwork we had filled out, we had not ticked the box beside "Alcohol or Drug abuse from Mother" in the Conditions of Acceptance form—this was a mandatory self-analysis form meant to gauge what we felt capable of responding to in terms of pre-existing challenges.

"That's right," I said.

"Not to discourage you, but you should know, sir, that ninety-five percent of the children we have in care face that challenge." I didn't know how to respond to this.

These were trying times, and difficult decisions and uncertainty abounded. Hope was doing great, and I could see her recovering, body and mind, from the crushing disappointment, the invasive procedures, and the progesterone shots—it's worth point out, by the way, that those painful progesterone shots had an oral alternative that the previous clinic never informed us of.

As an aside we had kept a picture of the embryo that had survived the longest. It seems random but it was the closest thing to being our baby who had actually being a living entity for some brief moments.

We were now ready to take a breath and re-group, hopeful at the thought of our upcoming appointment at the new clinic which promised a more caring, person-centred conversational approach.

It was kind of symbolic really. We were both looking at our occupations and moving towards places that were more aligned with ourselves. The biggest lesson we were learning was to trust our intuition much quicker than we'd been doing before.

Hope went to the new clinic and was able to go before work as it was much closer by. That evening, she recounted her experience which, as suspected, was worlds apart from the previous one. The doctor was on time and patient, as Hope recounted her story. The doctor asked for clarification where needed and patiently listened to the whole story. She then paged the receptionist for tissue and a glass of water for Hope and gave advice based on patients' experiential evidence both medical and non-medical. This doctor was insightful, patient and knowledgeable, and it made all the difference that she was also empathic, kind, and present. Hope felt a thousand times better at the thought of just attending this clinic.

Let this by a lesson to all who read this—if it doesn't feel right at the clinic, its atmosphere, ethos, or the way the staff treat you, then it isn't. Get out. Don't waste your time and energy.

Hope was advised to do a blood test that would actually tell her what her ovarian reserve was instead of basing it off anecdotal evidence from one IVF cycle. The doctor also recommended a supplement called royal jelly as it had been reported by a significant amount of successful patients (i.e. parents) to have made a difference. Apparently it's what the queen bee feasts on—I have no idea if that's true or not. Finally, the doctor also recommended an ultrasound and another sonohysterogram. Apparently the interpretations of these procedures are rather subjective, and she wanted to be able to use her own judgment before making any recommendations. The ultrasound was not a problem, but Hope had previously found the sonohysterogram so excruciatingly painful that we questioned whether it was completely necessary to do it again. We decided to try and see if the blood test and ultrasound would be enough data to get some significant feedback to inform any decisions without having to do another sonohysterogram.

Shortly after that initial consult, the doctor went on vacation for a few weeks, and in a way, it was probably good, for we really needed to take a break too. We booked a week off in the UK because of a wedding invitation from a close friend of mine. It was a chance to see my British family and, of course, to see my friend getting married. It was also a long overdue vacation.

It was only a week, and it was in the beginning of winter in a Northern hemisphere climate, yet we were so grateful to be able to regroup, relax, enjoy and find peace over the next little while to start afresh going into the New Year. It can be kind of great that life carries on when you've built yourself up so much for a moment that, in your mind, at the time, determines the course of your future. And in a way it does, but what influences it more so is your attitude to life's events.

In the meantime, other people around us were having babies. We were aunt and uncle to one niece already with another niece or nephew on the way. I started to mourn the idea of Hope being pregnant. I mean, I had always known I would need medical intervention to procreate, but it wasn't until we discovered how much trouble we'd have getting Hope pregnant that we realized how much we wanted it. I was mightily proud of how courageous she had been for fighting for something we wanted and was glad and privileged to be her partner. Now was the time to really reflect on what we *did* have rather than what we did not: a warm house, jobs, friends, family, food, relative safety, and hopeful futures. We kept focusing on that and used the final month of this long year to nurture our spirits and regain our strength and fortitude so that we could move into the New Year and face whatever 2015 had to offer.

Eighteen

THE LONG AND THE SHORT OF IT WAS THAT IT WAS coming towards the end of 2014. Our niece was growing, our friends around us all getting pregnant. We had tried so very hard and now did not know what to do. We had done some tests with the new clinic and had been asked to return for the results in January. In the meantime, we contacted the Children's Aid Society (CAS) again. We'd been told that one-and-a-half to two years *after* attending orientation we'd be in the process of training and then adoption ready. That was almost three and a half years ago, and despite our follow up calls and a promise that we'd get a call imminently, nothing surfaced. At this point we felt the need to just do something with these passing days. We called a few private adoption practitioners. We booked to go see someone for a consultation. It was just something else we could do, to at least gather more information.

Hope felt surges of anger at times, at how and why we would have to go through such an invasive process in order to adopt, including answering questions about our sex life and other issues from out past that other parents would never need face. Yes, CAS can ask you about all sorts of things. Other days, we were more accepting and would try and spin it in our heads as simply more good stuff for us to understand in terms of how to be better parents and be more self-aware and aware of each other's needs as we aged.

We met up with a couple of friends who'd adopted in another city. The same process there had taken only one year. They had given us the lowdown on the questions we might be asked. They'd already heard how shite the process was where we lived before.

We talked to a private practitioner and found out that in late 2014, Ontario had forty-seven separate, mostly-autonomous Children's Aid Societies, each with their sets of rules and regulations. A three-year wait just for *training* was not unusual for our local CAS. Furthermore, unlike other Children's Aid Societies, ours would not let us take our CAS assessment elsewhere in search of children requiring a home—even though this was common practice in all other Children's Aid Societies.

Thus the market for private practitioners such as the one we were talking to. You pay the practitioner around $2000 to do the training and the assessment and you own your assessment results and can take it to any other CAS in the province. We found out that twice a year all the Children's Aid Societies come to the Toronto Convention Centre and exhibit their hard-to-place children. This was also a chance for prospective adoptive parents to market themselves too.

The practitioner showed us books—we're talking glossy, professionally-bound—that adoptive parents had felt compelled created to showcase themselves and their current family make up and what they had to offer a child. It felt like bidding for a house against dozens if not hundreds of others. It was very surreal and more than a little unsettling. I must admit I felt momentarily excited at the thought of possibly welcoming a child into our lives by the end of the year. Then the thought of participating in what was effectively a child meat-market at the Toronto Convention Centre hit me square in the chest. Not the place for an introvert.

There were also websites of private adoption agencies with clients who create profiles of themselves for the benefit of birth parents who need to give their children up for adoption. If you are going to forgo the CAS and privately adopt, then you might want to have a look at these websites—just google them in your area. This usually involves a young person, often religious, who is either unable or unwilling (or both) to consider abortion. They have approached a private adoption agency to have their unexpected child adopted *at birth*. The practitioner informed us that there were less than a hundred babies adopted this way each year in Ontario.

After our meeting with the private practitioner, Hope and I decided that of the two options in front of us—IVF and adoption—adoption was not so time sensitive. So again, we came back to waiting for the results from the clinic on the blood tests to understand our antral follicle (ovarian reserve) count.

IN THE MEANTIME, I WAS THINKING ABOUT MY LIFE every day. My daily routine was: get up, get ready, go to work, work, eat lunch, work more, go to the gym, go home, eat dinner, chill out, go to bed. That was basically my life. I would find it boring most of the time at best. I would have to remind myself how incredibly *fortunate* I was to be able to be bored because I was safe, housed, clothed, fed and loved.

And don't get me wrong, I did *not* want to have a child in order to alleviate boredom. I started to think that I was shutting down that part of my brain that got excited about life because it was too overwhelming to think that, well, *this was it.* This was all life had to offer me. I don't mean that I didn't love the people in my life and they weren't enough; of course, they were. I think maybe at times I might also have romanticized having a child. What helped me have faith that we could do it was the fact that Hope worked with children every day, and although she was always—and I do mean *always* exhausted—she was also always satisfied by the profoundness of impacting young people's critical development and watching them grow. She would come home with stories of how a child had started to understand things like the process of tidying up independently, or colour changes, or sharing for example. It would be amazing to hear.

I would tell Hope, that since our child/children are not here, we could try and enjoy life in other ways, such as going out to eat more, or try to bring joy in different ways into the world. I started volunteering for a charity that gives respite to families with children with autism. I also would see on my sister-in-law's face at times the exhaustion of having children, and recognized that I didn't have that. I could sleep, eat, and do what I wanted *when* I wanted. We would often hear folks who had young kids tell us that we don't realize how selfish we are until children come. I took that to mean that basic needs like peeing by yourself on your own time is a luxury when you are a parent of a young one.

In the meantime, we bounced back and forth each day trying to manage our emotions. We'd decided that we wouldn't be doing anything until these test results came through in January, and in a way, that gave us permission to enjoy a bit of a break until then. And I think we both needed that.

TIME PASSED. PEOPLE'S LIVES CONTINUED. MORE friends had more babies.

That Christmas we were surrounded by family from all generations, including the emerging life in the belly of my younger sister-in-law. I could appreciate that those people who cared for us—and wished us nothing but success—were at times perhaps feeling complicated about celebrating and enjoying their imminent life changes in front of us. It can be ticklish. We would spend time drilling home the message that we could and *did* love and enjoy other's celebratory moments of new life as it was quite healing—because we *chose* to see it that way.

When I found myself getting angry at the situation—usually tied up with the feeling of not being in control which was in turn tied to other baggage—my goal was to recognize the anger and channel that energy into as positive a drive as I could. I would strive to validate how hard we had fought and what an amazing experience it was. I would be thankful for everything I had (including the freedom that comes from not having kids), and I would try to move forward.

On Christmas morning Hope and I exchanged our gifts under the tree. One of my gifts to Hope was a $15,000 signed cheque from me to her as a symbol to try another IVF cycle at some point into the future. I think we had both intuitively known that, at some point, we were going to be doing this again, now that we had made some positive changes in our lives to reduce the stress and optimize the good spirited energy around us.

First of all, we were both exercising more, and my new job situation was a lot more conducive to my own values. Secondly, we had switched clinics and the philosophy of the new place was phenomenally different from the previous place. In fact, it was so different that I felt compelled to write a letter to our former fertility clinic listing all of the processes that we had experienced there. I tried to write it as objectively as possible. Suffice to say that was rather therapeutic.

OUR NEW YEAR'S GOALS INCLUDED MOVING towards what we *did* want by getting rid of what we *didn't* want. This included a professional organizer coming in to help us clear out our clutter. We felt lighter and reinvigorated, and visualizing new ventures felt easier. We started to discuss investment opportunities and began planning as though these children were *going* to come.

I started my volunteering for a local charity that helps children with autism. We helped our local church go through a formal process of become more affirming and welcoming to the LGBT [lesbian gay bisexual transgendered] community. For me, giving out more was helpful and kept me from focusing so much on the empty holes in my own life. It reminding me of what I *did* have. In fact, within the first month of the New Year I found myself unexpectedly doing resuscitation on a toddler who collapsed at a bus stop on the sidewalk near my workplace. I was relieved to discover this child regained consciousness later in hospital, and it made me think of the terrible awfulness of losing a child—it is almost beyond comprehension.

Keeping busy helped pass the time.

WHEN HOPE'S RESULTS FROM THE NEW CLINIC CAME back they showed she was indeed completely average for her age in terms of her antral follicle count. This really sealed the deal in our minds. We *were* going to try IVF again at some point. In terms of timing, our thoughts bounced around all over the place. Obviously, like most folks, we were balancing between wanting to do it as soon as possible—time was of the essence—but also saving up enough to avoid a precarious financial position. There was also the consideration of whether we were in the absolute best condition physically and emotionally, optimizing our chances by eating better, sleeping better, exercising more and being kinder to ourselves.

All these considerations aside, our spirits were high.

As the weeks passed, we decided to explore new housing developments in our area as an option to invest money to finance our expensive journey. Of course we were just dreaming at this point, but the information we gathered taught us pretty quickly what we could and couldn't afford. We were considering of downsizing to an apartment to be able to pay for IVF funding. It was early March 2015 and IVF was still not a funded procedure.

In early March, my mother came for a visit just as the GTA was hit with a massive power outage that left of 25,000 in the dark. A terrible storm had loaded power lines down with ice, and when lines started falling, transformers started going up. Temperatures plunged and many folks were left without power for up to a week. I was a tad concerned, but at the same time too emotionally exhausted to care too much. I was actually starting to question how much I felt about anything.

A couple of days later, we had a big family dinner, and our elders shared with us their experiences of home ownership. From the wisdom I could hear, they were encouraging us to consider carefully why we were considering a move and what other options we might have to stay. They encouraged us to think carefully about the issues at play. It was a helpful discussion mainly in that it helped me realize that I was becoming emotionally dissociated. I no longer knew how I truly felt about the house, the idea of moving, the idea of paying to try to make a baby again. It was all getting a bit overwhelming. We had already been through a lot. We both needed a break to be able to get some space away from everything and not even think too much about these topics.

We talked about trying in May and having a substantial vacation immediately after the transfer attempt. That meant the end of May early June for that vacation, but of course, trying to book a vacation for the day after the transfer without *knowing* the date of the transfer was next to impossible, and this inevitably tweaked my need to feel in control again. Maybe it would be better to stick around for a guaranteed period of time to ensure we were here for the monitoring of the situation when we tried again then follow *that* with a vacation.

It would either be a celebratory vacation or a consolatory one where we would have to reflect on decisions moving forward with family making. Either way, it was going to require some time out together away from all other concerns.

Nineteen

AS APRIL ROLLED AROUND, THE FINAL COUNTDOWN to my younger sister-in-law's due date was fast approaching. We had a family Easter dinner, and at that point the poor woman just felt physically uncomfortable and was more than ready to pop this kid out already! Both Hope and I felt a great excitement to meet this child as we had with our first niece. Meanwhile life continued to push us in the direction it wanted us to go in, which was not what we'd predicted. Hope found herself possibly in line for a significant promotion. A huge opportunity. Of course, being the authentic person she is, Hope immediately thought about how she'd only be in this new position for nine months if she got pregnant finally in May and how that would impact the company. I tried to remind her that people who get pregnant naturally don't think like this—life just *happens* in its own unpredictable manner. I even tried to put it to her that perhaps that would even be a good thing e.g., she could lay down the foundations of the position before someone takes over once she is on leave.

We'd left our next clinic attempt until May due to predictable stressors, and now life was reminding us yet again that it was nothing if not unpredictable! We needed to stop trying to manage things so much. Because we had our sights set on May, the new clinic had wanted us to contact them in April.

Well, here we were.

This clinic, as I have mentioned, was way more in line with our values and had brought Hope far more peace in mind, body and spirit than the previous one. An ultrasound was booked for late April, as was a mandatory education session that was anticipated to be up to an hour and a half. Part of me was skeptical.

Oh come on. At this point what the fuck can they possibly tell us about this process that we don't know already?

But part of me was also intrigued, particularly as they knew our circumstances and history. It had to be booked during working hours, but I was going to do my best to attend this with Hope.

I have to say, this clinic was very receptive and communicative. Now you might think that *all* clinics would be like this, but you'd be wrong. The first notable difference was that doctors themselves responded to emails directly from the patient. What a concept! The alleviation of anxiety this brought for us both was immense, which of course was all the more conducive to staying relaxed, calm and comfortable, which in turn optimized the chances of success. They had also recommended several options *outside* the strict realm of medicine such as supplements and exercises for both mind and body. Hope was practicing yoga, meditation, and reading incredibly helpful books that were taking a more holistic approach to a woman's fertility.

The themes were all about reflecting on the person's relation-ship with femininity, receptive energy, and how historically its meaning and people's perception of it has been skewed in many cultures as dirty, bad, wrong and shameful. There was a lot of time spent unlearning all the negative messages that were so deeply rooted and accepting the feminine and what that actually meant. I spoke with my female peers and friends and found this more and more common. I explored articles and writings of women's attempts to take back and learn to appreciate that feminine can mean strength and integrity and be nurturing and empowering in many ways. The bottom line message was about being receptive without being submissive while at the same time not vilifying submissiveness in and of itself—something too often occurring in the media.

The take away message for me was this: support your partner in whichever way they self-identify. Not just their gender identity or other feelings they have, but how they see themselves in different mental and emotional states. If your partner feels like they do not like how their body works, for instance, this is an area that could be a great opportunity for the support person to help. Try and invite your partner to consider that this part of her body is divine, that the body is doing what needs to happen in order for life to be sustainable. That it is this miraculous process happening within them where the phenomenon of new life emerges. Try to use sincere yet empowering words. Be sure to acknowledge their very real thoughts and feelings whatever they are. In a nutshell meet them where they are and carefully encourage them to accept that this is *life* happening within them—how they choose to respond to it is up to them. If you see or hear *any* messages in the media or from friends that are reinforcing the idea of shame in any way around the feminine, call it out immediately. You want to essentially act as an ally for your partner's body. Love their body as the house of their soul. Their body is the house of your baby's first nine months of life.

Okay, I know. Here endeth the lesson. Anyway, back to the clinic.

THEY DID NOT HAVE TO DO TOO MUCH TO IMPRESS US
after the previous experience we had endured. Direct email communications and a phone line to the lead nurse to quell any anxieties from a medical standpoint was very helpful. Their policy was for the prospective patient to give them a heads up a month in advance of the cycle and also a $250 deposit. It was helpful to keep us going because there were many apprehension moments. Those are moments when you suddenly have a bit of an anxiety attack and question what you are doing.

Twenty thousand dollars?! For a less than a fifty-fifty chance? That's nuts. I could travel to see Europe from North America twelve times over for that kind of money! I could likely build a small housing establishment in a village in Burkina Faso for that money... I could...

One thing that I think helped me was reminding myself that I was comparing my procreation situation to that of folks who could conceive naturally. This was something I often caught myself doing and always had to give my head a shake. I recall conversations about how this self-comparison was not helpful because then the inevitable feelings of it being *unfair* would flood my mind and overwhelm me. Then of course, after being overwhelmed, a sense of depression would set in. I realized around this time—and understand that it had taken me a *long* time to get there—that all I have control over is how I *respond* to these intrusive thoughts and feelings.

Haruki Murakami, in his book *What I Talk About When I Talk About Running*, quotes a mantra he heard from another runner.

"Pain is inevitable. Suffering is optional."

WHEN I STARTED THINKING ABOUT MY TRIGGERS and responses, I was able to start to defuse the anxiety around the inevitable apprehension moments and stop driving myself nuts. It helped me slow things down and learn to appreciate the authenticity of the relationships in my life—my relationship with Hope, with family, friends, and myself and my relationship with my yet-to-be-conceived child.

Twenty

ONE OF THE SUGGESTIONS OF THE NEW CLINIC WAS that we change *everything*—the donor, the drugs, the approach, all of it. There was something appealing about that. When it came to the donor, we discovered that we now had to pay two hundred dollars for an account if we wanted to view the donors' written essays. We could review the pertinent stats of a donor (health status, family history, nostril hair length, etc.) for free, but we wanted to know a bit about the individuals as people, the energy of the donor that was going to be part of making this potential child. Two hundred dollars. Can you say cash grab?

Furthermore, since the last time we had been on the donor site, the donor list had changed significantly. There were a few folks left on there that we had reviewed before, but a lot had accounts less than a month old. We embarked on reading the essays of new donors. As before, we narrowed things down by filtering for donors with similar physical attribute to myself. I believe this left something like a hundred and eight profile essays to read.

Eventually I started to see the theme in how these essays were formatted. They would start with a structure of brief early childhood, family background, school life, interests, sports, career choices, outlook on life, and their personal message to the potential child. I started to just read the last paragraph, i.e. their outlook and message to the child. That to me was the most important part of the donor's energy. It did not take too long to make the donor choice.

"be who you are [and] *...don't ever lose sight of the true joy of life and accept yourself and others."*

Sounds a bit wishy washy as I write it here now, partly because I cannot fully recall it to hand, but it was very much in line with what we would want our child (or children) to hear daily. We'd wanted them to know that they were loved, that they were meant to be here, and that the most important thing was to be at peace with who they are.

We were happy with our choice.

The next step of course was to pay the $250 deposit for the cycle. I understood why it was important. Providers needed to prepare for staffing arrangements and so on. We made the deposit right around the time Hope was offered her big job opportunity, and that coincidence felt very much like life was sending us a message of some sort—but what *was* the message? Was it that something is *always* going to come up? Or was it that maybe now was not quite the right time to try after all?

There were three possible courses of action.

First, Hope could turn down the opportunity, fearing that the inevitable stress could have an impact on her ability to conceive and knowing that, if successful, her pregnancy would force her to give up the new position in nine months' time. Alternatively, she could take the job and pursue the procedure anyway, letting the chips fall where they may. And finally we could decide to delay our next attempt until she was settled into the new job things weren't so stressful.

The forty-eight hours following the job was offered was a bit of a rollercoaster.

To be honest, the most compelling argument against the last course of action was that we had already paid the $250 deposit and would lose it if we cancelled. However, $250 in the grand scheme of $20,000 is really not that big of a deal. After much hemming and hawing, we decided to delay. Emails with the nurse confirmed that, yes, we'd lose the $250, but she agreed that perhaps the decision was for the best all things considered.

She also share with us how cruel she thought it was that the provincial government had not come through with more details on their promised IVF coverage—we thought so too. It had been a year since the Ontario Health Minister, committed to a 2015 rollout, but the ministry not shared any information with clinics and it was already April. Furthermore, the nurse advised us to not rely on this happening any time soon because once details were finally rolled out it would take time for policies and procedures to be put in place. We got the message that if we wanted to optimize our chances of this IVF cycle working, it would be best to pay privately for it so that it happens sooner rather than later.

Still, we decided to delay. It was a tough call, but we felt it was the right one. It would only be for a few months. No longer than that. Time enough for Hope to settle into her new job, for us to adjust our diets, look more into fertility health outside of medical systems, and improve our general well-being. There was also the matter of when we could take time off, post-embryo transfer as required for the IVF process. We decided on September 2015. Four months. A third of a year.

I was happy to just accept this, loosen my death grip on the (mostly imaginary) reins of control, and give up the idea that we could somehow eliminate the element chance from the equation. The sole element of control I felt was the money I had managed to save up over the past five years. Saving money had become not only a habit but a displacement activity for all the things I could not control.

Who knew what the future held? I sure as hell didn't. All I knew was that I had opened my bank account regularly to see that money sitting in there, not *doing* anything. I had considered investment opportunities to try and put the money to work, but I didn't like the risk or the thought of tying any of it up. And to be honest—and this is where I kept coming back to—what else was I actually going to spend this money on?

I was not going to go on a $20,000 trip. I had travelled the world and found a sense of profound emptiness until I had discovered myself through falling in love with someone who helped me accept myself. A $20,000 down-payment on another property? I knew myself, and I would only find that taking over my days and nights, my thoughts and emotional energy—and to what end? I was determined to stay focussed and in the moment, as the support partner for what Hope and I were going through that was the least I could do.

Not that investing in property is not a good idea. I think it is actually a very smart idea, but it's not entirely without risk (and thus stress) and demands at least some of your attention.

No, I knew, now more than ever, that there was nothing else I wanted to spend that money on. And losing our deposit and deciding on September (regardless of provincial funding that might never materialize) felt affirming. This was going to be our shot.

We would eat healthy, treat ourselves, live a little, enjoy the summer, and settle into our new routines.

Twenty-one

IN APRIL MY SECOND NIECE WAS ENJOYING A COZY nine extra days beyond her due date in the comfort of her mother's womb before she was born. Hope and I had the privilege of meeting her the night she was born. What an amazing experience. It felt so awesome to have not just the three generations in the same room again, but three sisters hovering over this child. Let me just say that Hope comes from a long line of strong women, so I felt pretty confident that this new one in the room was going to be just fine! It is such an incredible thing to witness a newborn adjusting to air and people. And it is an amazing experience having the calmness coming over everyone who is around them. It is one of those experiences in life that makes everyone, no matter where they are at in their lives, stop and step back and look around at the world because it will never be the same place again now that this new life is in it.

Both Hope and I got to hold our new niece that night. I felt so serene inside to be holding her—all the other dramas and difficulties of my life dissolved into nothingness. This energy was what was important to me.

Some friends and family members were a little concerned, given the difficulties Hope and I had been through trying to conceive, about how it would feel watching another family member have a child. But it could not have been more comforting. I am not sure how you might react, but there was only love pouring out of both of our hearts for this new family addition. That night, we went for an evening stroll back to our car as we left the hospital and knew implicitly that this child had encouraged us to try just one more time.

WE SAW A NATUROPATH AND STARTED MAKING more and more dietary changes that were clearly having positive effects on both of our moods and bodies. We explored other supports in different towns and even countries. We skyped a fertility naturopath in California for advice on immunology and fertility issues. This was also a learning journey for me. We discovered that subclinical thyroid issues are only explored if one overarching hormone, TSH [thyroid-stimulating hormone], is outside the normal range. However, it controls a whole cascade of processes and sub-steps that, if not measured, make it hard to tell what is really going on. Consider looking into this if you can if it seems relevant to you. Several blood tests were called for to confirm, before and after dietary changes, what might be going on. And we discovered that the thyroid was definitely sluggish. So Hope cut out gluten as advised by the naturopath Apparently, gluten can act like an irritant in the gut and behave similarly to thyroxine, the hormone controlling metabolism in the body (well, one hormone of many). The recommendation was to now cut out dairy, too, as well as caffeine and red meat.

I wanted to try and show Hope solidarity as much as I could. I was at the same time going through my own body-changing goals of putting on more mass, and red meat was a big option for that!

But we found that, like any habit, changing our diets got easier and easier each day until we no longer missed bread or yoghurt. I could also see us becoming calmer and more peaceful. The quality of sleep improved as well. We felt less sluggish and more comfortable in our bodies in general. I knew that, no matter what, , I was happy to see increased health in general.

We had certainly learned that Western medicine and naturopathic medicine were very much parallel opposites in their approach to the patient. Naturopath doctors were far more empowering in general and inclined to work *with* the body rather than going so quickly to medications to replace and substitute the body's own functions. I do not want to put medicine or medications down as I myself rely on them for functions my body is missing, and we were certainly going to need Western medicine for the IVF cycle. My main point here is to be open-minded to other approaches if one is not necessarily fitting too well with your needs.

That was the other great aspect of our new fertility clinic and fertility specialist: they were working with the findings of our naturopath, and because of these changes, they recommended that we hold off for a period of time before trying. We chose to wait until November 2015 before trying IVF again. That way we would have enough time for these positive changes to take maximum effect on the eggs that were currently maturing inside Hope's ovaries.

It is important to know that the quality of your lifestyle now, will impact the eggs your partner will ovulate in three to six months' time. We both saw this as a chance to feel as fully empowered as possible before trying, so we agreed to this.

That summer my mum came to stay with us for seven weeks. Because we would now not be gearing up for our next attempt during her visit, it enabled us to enjoy the summer with her and one of my brothers who was between leaving his job in China and starting his new job in Dubai.

THE FALL CAME AND WAS A TIME OF CHANGE AND not just in the weather. With my mum and brother gone, I realized I needed to prioritize my relationship with Hope more significantly. Hope and I went through what almost could be likened to a performance appraisal of where we were with our relationship. Four key principles were reviewed: communication, intimacy, trust and acceptance. We asked each other to consider own ideal states of what these looked like in a relationship and then what they actually did look like in their current states. We then compared notes and it evoked conversations and helped highlight the gaps between us. Those gaps enabled us to come up with some specific actions to try to ensure we were as solid as we could be as we geared up for one last attempt at conception. We were pleased to discover that we both had an almost identical wording for our definition of an ideal relationship. That's always a plus.

I felt very lucky to have such a wonderful partner with her perspective and balance helping me to stay grounded. I started journaling and sharing the journal with Hope who also tried to write in her thoughts and feelings. It was helpful.

We were approaching November and as it got closer and closer all those wild and wonderful doubts were building up. At one point in October, as we were getting ready to contact the clinic and put down a new deposit, Hope texted me in the morning from work asking if I thought we should wait to see if the government would fund by the end of the year—it was October after all—or go for it. I pointed out that, current promises aside, the government had been saying they were going to fund IVF cycles for over eight years and that, given how time sensitive our chances were, we should take it into our own hands.

It's now or never, I thought. *It's fear-based thinking to wait. It's empowering to grasp the bull by the horns...*

She agreed.

Three hours later—I am not kidding—the government made a public announcement that they had finally made it official that funding would begin in December.

Arrrgh!

My initial thought when I heard this was that is too good to be true, which was Hope's thoughts too. To make a long story short, this is something like how the next two weeks went right up to the decision day:

"Wow! Good job we were going to wait until November, it means that we were on the verge of paying $20,000, but now if we wait one extra month we can use that money for so many other things."

"Hang on a second, our clinic won't do cycles in December, so that would make it January. January in Canada is very difficult to travel in with the snow and cold and dark."

"On the other hand, if we do it in January and it doesn't work, then we have $20,000 to put towards private adoption as public adoption has not followed through with us at all."

"But what will happen to the wait lists now that access will increase? People who normally wouldn't even consider IVF due to the expense will be flocking to the clinics, our clinic has told us there would be no special privileges given to people who had already been with the clinic."

"True, and if we wait, we will be competing with others not just for the actual IVF cycle treatment, but also for the daily cycle monitoring which will be very stressful."

"But if it doesn't work we will have lost $20,000."

"But if we don't try and have to wait for a long time to be seen, and it *fails*, we'll always wonder what would have happened if we'd acted sooner. And our legacy will be that we waited because of the money."

WE TALKED ABOUT IT A GREAT DEAL, WEIGHING THE pros against cons as the calendar crept towards the day we'd need to place our deposit—decision day. It was helpful to focus on how the government had restricted the IVF funded cycle to only one embryo transfer process regardless of how many embryos you may produce and freeze, whereas our own funded cycle would allow for two embryos to be transfered if we wanted, which we did. Our clinic, we knew, wouldn't prioritize people who were be willing to pay over those government funded, which meant that November would be the final month of our lives that we would be able to try under the current circumstances. November meant doing it on our own terms, non-funded, but our way, if we were ready—which we were.

We called up the clinic and made our deposit.

When we were ready to order the donor units we discovered that there was only one unit left—not that the procedure required more than one. This meant that, after the current attempt, if it failed and we decided to pursue a government funded attempt, it would have to be with a different donor. We reviewed the other donors from whom more than one unit remained, and in the end we just felt right with our first choice. We knew that it would be a possibility to have more than one embryo out of one IVF cycle with one unit—it all depended on the quality of eggs that were retrieved. Ultimately, quality was more important than quantity, and quality was heavily dependent on age, so we felt the optimal time to try was now.

We had gotten ourselves into a good headspace. We'd changed jobs, were eating better, taking supplements, receiving acupuncture (shown anecdotally to help with fertility), listening to fertility meditation programs every night, going for massage treatments, and feeling more in control. We were sticking with our one-unit donor, and we were going to go for it.

Now it was a matter of settling as comfortably into the situation as possible and contemplating how we were going to be able to move on with our lives if this didn't work. We were realistic this time, talking about that possibility rather than being afraid to mention it at all. And we both agreed that, when it comes right down to it, we'd rather regret something we'd done than something we hadn't done.

For fun, we consulted a psychic and were told that November was showing as month of conception, learning of a pregnancy, or of a baby's birth—which suggested that IVF in November would appear to coincide with this psychic's sense. Whatever you happen to think about the Law of Attraction, I think it's helpful, at the very least, to have a clear vision of what it is you hope to achieve.

Twenty-two

EVERYTHING WAS IN PLACE. WE COULD NOT HAVE been more ready, focussed or determined. We went to the clinic to initiate the procedures we knew so well. The monitoring, the drugs, pills and injections, the blood tests, the progress updates, the scheduling of the optimal moment for triggering. All the while we were more at peace than during previous attempts because we could see that this had been a true journey of facing our fears and the recognizing the meaning we had given to our lives and our trek up to this point. The doctor was calm and the nurses and staff were kind. The space was more spa-like and even the sun was shining in the crisp and clear mornings when we had to go for a follow up blood test—which would not likely have been the case in January.

We went in for the egg retrieval, we knew the drill. Although at last count a set number of eggs were assessed as maturing, a call back later that day revealed, rather than via a neon sign in the room, that despite efforts to increase Hope's number of eggs, only five eggs had been made and were retrieved. It felt like a door was slowly closing.

The next day the news was sobering. Only four of the five eggs had successfully fertilized. Again, it felt as though the lights were being turned off with only a candle in the middle of the room still lit.

The following day we were told that only two of the four fertilized eggs were still alive and growing, so the clinic urged us to come in for a day-three transfer. The candle was burning low.

The day of the transfer, moments before the procedure, we were told there was only one fertilized egg left and that it was only six cells rather than the eight to ten the clinic would have preferred. The egg was implanted. The candle flame was guttering.

WE HAD BOOKED A TRIP TO SAN FRANCISCO TO PASS the two week wait before we could test for pregnancy, and spent mid-December walking the hills of that remarkable city. And for the first time in a *very* long time, we really enjoyed the present moment. We visited ancient redwood forests, took in the city parks, sampled terrific seafood, and caught up with a couple of folks who lived in the state. We explored the bay and Japan town—which reminded us of Japan where we had first met all those years ago.

While we were in California, Hope administered daily progesterone suppositories as advised by the clinic, and the day finally arrived when we could actually test for the results. In fact, that day both came and *went*, for we decided to wait until we got back to Canada to know our fate, keeping the hope of not knowing alive at least until the end of our trip.

We got back on a weekend and Hope's blood test was scheduled for first thing Monday morning. We could have purchased a pee-stick from Walmart, of course, but we didn't.

The morning the alarm went off at six o'clock. Hope did her usual morning routine and set off for the clinic a portrait of calm. The usual call from the clinic—on Hope's phone—came a few hours later, but we decided, not to listen to it until we were together in the evening after work.

As I finished an otherwise-typical Monday at work, I was praying and hoping—knowing the inevitable was coming. Already I was thinking what might I do to support Hope when the candle finally burns out?

We arrived home and hugged.

There was no voice mail from the clinic. How could they not leave a message and put us out of our misery at least?

Then, an email arrived from the clinic with a single word in the subject line: Results.

Hope, unable to read it, asked me to instead.

I opened the email and saw lots of writing. I scrolled down.

"Oh my God, Hope!"

"What?"

"Oh my God... you're pregnant.

CPSIA information can be obtained
at www.ICGtesting.com
Printed in the USA
LVHW090104300319
612423LV00016B/503/P

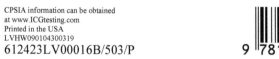

9 781460 297964